C000092980

MY HEALTH UPGRADED

REVOLUTIONARY TECHNOLOGIES TO BRING A HEALTHIER FUTURE

BERTALAN MESKO

Publisher: Webicina Kft.
My Health: Upgraded
Revolutionary Technologies To Bring A Healthier Future
Bertalan Mesko

Copyright © 2015 by Dr. Bertalan Mesko
All rights reserved.

Editor: Dr. Richard E. Cytowic
Cover Design: Roland Rekeczki
Interior Design: Roland Rekeczki
Illustrations: Richard Horvath

This book was self–published by the author under Webicina Kft. No part of this book may be reproduced in any form by any means without the express permission of the author. This includes reprints, excerpts, photocopying, recording, or any future means of reproducing text.

If you would like to do any of the above or need information on bulk purchases, please contact the author at http://www.medicalfuturist.com and info@the-medicalfuturist.com.

ISBN 978–615–80261–0–9 (paperback)
ISBN 978–615–80261–1–6 (e–book)

Printed by CreateSpace, An Amazon.com Company.
Printed in the United States of America.

References appear at the end of the book.

The content of this book is for informational purposes only and does not constitute professional medical advice, legal advice, diagnosis, treatment or recommendation of any specific treatment or provider of any kind. Individuals should always seek the advice of qualified professionals with any questions or concerns about their health or treatment. Neither the author nor any of the content in this book is meant to recommend or endorse specific hospitals, physicians, cities, hotels, facilities, or procedures. We advise readers to do their own research and due diligence, make their own informed decisions and seek their own medical and legal advice. Reliance on any information provided in this book is solely at your own risk.

TABLE OF CONTENTS

ABOUT THE AUTHOR

Dr. Bertalan Mesko, PhD is a medical futurist who gives presentations at institutions including the World Health Organization and Yale, Stanford, and Harvard universities on how to establish a mutually positive relationship between the human touch and innovative technologies. He is the author of The Guide to the Future of Medicine, featured in Amazon's top 100 books. He is a medical doctor with a PhD in genomics.

One of the world's leading biotech thinkers, Dr. Mesko serves as a consultant for pharmaceutical and medical technology companies. He works to educate health care professionals on how to use disruptive technologies effectively to converse with patients. He is the managing director and founder of Webicina, the first service that curates the medical and health-related social media resources for patients and medical professionals.

His work has been featured by CNN, the World Health Organization, National Geographic, Forbes, TIME, BBC, the New York Times, and Wired Science among others.

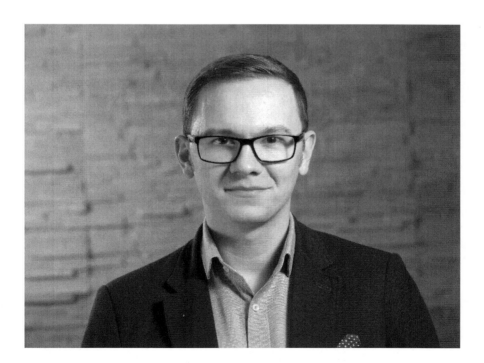

ADVANCED PRAISE FOR MY HEALTH: UPGRADED

"Dr. Bertalan Mesko, the consummate medical futurist, takes us on an extended technological tour - one that bodes well for how healthcare can advance."
- Dr. Eric Topol, author of The Patient Will See You Now, Professor of Genomics, The Scripps Research Institute

"Dr. Bertalan Mesko has been called a thought leader thanks to his views on the future of medicine, and his latest book proves yet again just why he deserves that title. Dr. Mesko's thoughts on digital health are comprehensive and innovative, but most importantly, they are accessible and easily understood. This thrilling book is a must-read for patients, providers, and all other stakeholders interested in taking control of their own health."
- Dr. Larry Chu, Executive Director, Stanford Medicine X

"Sit down, loosen your mind, and settle into this book. It's an extraordinary, liberated tour of what health and treatment will be like when we no longer starve for information and when everything physical is digital - which is far closer than you think."
- e-Patient Dave deBronkart, e-patient thought leader, speaker, author

"Only few have the gift of being transformative ·nd using it; Dr. Bertalan Mesko is one of them. This book bridges Hype, Hope & reality in a way that fits both the world of technology and medicine. Definitely a must read if you're on the intersection of technology & medicine."
- Lucien Engelen, Director of the Radboud REshape Innovation Center

"An easy to read guide to future health. Introducing recent history and everyday examples of progress as evidence of trends, it looks to the future of health technologies and their interactions with everyday lifestyle with informed optimism, avoiding unnecessary jargon. Covering areas from personal health recording to cheap DNA sequencing and AI assistance, it shows how the reader can take control of their own health and the many future opportunities for improving it. It also explores when we will get the technologies we see in sci-fi movies. All of this makes it a compelling but easy-going read."
- Ian Pearson, Futurologist, Author of You Tomorrow

"Dr. Bertalan Mesko has written an amazingly interesting book that explores the future of medicine and how it will affect our health. As a transhumanist and politician, I highly recommend this book to all those who are interested in how technology is going to impact our bodies and change our lives."
- Zoltan Istvan, futurist and US Presidential candidate

"Three in one, My Health: Upgraded is a didactic snapshot of digital health today and to come, a practical "how-to" guide on self-tracking, and responses to real "questions from the audience". And Dr. Bertalan Mesko dares to answer them all. While I see many digital health books and articles, My Health:Upgraded is definitely not to be missed!"
- Denise Silber, Founder of Doctors 2.0 and You

"This one is just fantastic, an encyclopedic work by one of the recognized experts. No need to "Google" about the future of medicine, this book is like a search-engine on itself, about the amazing facts & possibilities of our health, but upgraded!"
- Dr. Rafael J. Grossmann, FACS, Surgeon, Healthcare Futurist & Innovator

INTRODUCTION

The technological revolution has posed big questions. What is the purpose of the human race? Can we retain the human touch in medicine while at the same time embracing disruptive innovations? Should we upgrade our health with ever–advancing technologies? Shall we keep our distance from artificial intelligence or robotics used in healthcare?

News every day makes us feel as if we live in a science fiction world. Exoskeletons let paralyzed people walk again. Algorithms diagnose medical conditions. The wearable revolution and a swarm of new sensors offer society amazing advantages but create risks we have never had to think of before. All this, and yet there are still many areas on earth where no care is delivered at all.

If we don't improve our skills and creativity, then robots and software will not only get better at doing our jobs but also render digital care without human interaction or empathy. The future we desire most should not be determined by technology, but by our chance to live healthily in freedom. It won't happen without us taking concrete steps. We should work harder to demonstrate why the human brain is the most complex object in the universe.

Rising healthcare costs in the face of decreasing quality of care should lead to the use of more and better technologies than what we have now. I hope to persuade you that we can make healthcare accessible and affordable worldwide, and to show that the road to it is paved with disruptive technologies. I'll further illustrate how technology can increase empathy, the human touch, and the doctor–patient relationship.

Good innovations can bring us closer to one another and in fact foster aspects that make us human. And yet some people will be skeptical and resist them. People might be excited about improvements in television, cars, or online services. But when it comes to health, even simple questions are difficult to answer. Will new radiology devices result in better prevention? Can the information in our DNA reliably predict future health? Who is allowed to access such information? These are the kinds of challenges that the technological revolution will present us in the coming years.

Starting in the 1990s, we went from watching movies on VHS cassettes, listening to music on CDs, and accessing a dial–up Internet connection via a desktop computer; to watching, listening to, and accessing digital data anywhere, anytime, on any device. We went from Walkmans to iTunes and Spotify. From videocameras to smartphones recording anything around us. From shopping in person to finding almost anything online. From printed encyclopedias to Wikipedia. From meeting friends in person to sharing what we see via virtual reality devices on Facebook. These kinds of changes took nearly two decades. The next replacements will overtake existing technology in months. And then the change will be measured in weeks or even days.

The technological revolution behind medicine has been huge. Hundreds of thousands have access to their genetic data that reveal what medical conditions they are susceptible to or what mutations they carry. Sensors in wearable devices let us measure vital signs and health parameters at home. Surgical robots have become more precise than ever, and increasingly human–looking robots are walking the floors of health clinics worldwide.

An Internet connection can bring medical expertise to areas that lack practitioners. Biotechnology can help us understand the body's microbiomes, or stimulate immune cells that fight tumors. Over the last few decades new drugs have been abundant and have improved lives by better managing diseases like diabetes and high blood pressure. Yet even though technology is improving at an incredible pace, it still manages to feel obsolete within a short time.

The technological revolution has been exploding, but the practice of medicine has made only small steps toward improved care. It seemed to be working well for the past hundred years, but not anymore. If we do not change how healthcare adjusts to the ever changing needs of patients and the opportunities that technology can deliver, it will lapse into chaos where human interaction has little or no value.

PART I. THE TECHNOLOGICAL REVOLUTION IN MEDICINE

The Case For Disruptive Innovations

Millions of medical studies and papers exist, making it humanly impossible for physicians to remain current without digital help. Some estimate that starting in 2020, the amount of medical data will double every 73 days. During their life an average individual will generate more than 1 million gigabytes of health–related data. Data sets that large can no longer be analyzed by people. Cognitive computers such as IBM's Watson can analyze tens of thousands of clinical studies and patient records, and suggest–for a particular patient–possible diagnoses and therapy options from which the physician can then choose. The time saved by crunching this enormous amount of data could be spent on direct patient care.

Radiology devices will soon provide real–time and more detailed images of a patient's internal organs. Virtual– and augmented reality devices will further improve this. Such images could help surgeons plan their operations more precisely by guiding 3D printers to produce models of a tumor or other abnormality. Such printers could also create economical prosthetics and instruments.

Patients can not receive proper medical care if they are unable to wear devices that monitor their vital signs and health parameters at home. Telemedicine services like this are vitally needed in areas that have a shortage of doctors. Without it, care cannot be delivered, patients must miss time from work, or travel to an institution far away. Biotechnology that can produce artificial organs in the lab could eliminate transplantation waiting lists forever. Virtual models could test potential new drugs in seconds instead of having to rely on lengthy and expensive clinical trials with real people as we do now.

New technologies are disruptive and revolutionary because they are less expensive, faster, and more efficient than previous ones.

For example, in the 1980s an electronic set of the Encyclopaedia Britannica cost about $2000. Physically it was big. Each of its two dozen volumes had an update cycle of at least a year. Now Wikipedia is free, accessible to anyone, and is updated constantly. Between 2003 and 2013 the price of flash memory found in USB drives dropped dramatically from $0.25 per megabyte to $0.0003, a change of three orders of magnitude in 10 years. Early 3D printers produced fairly low–quality products and took hours to do so.

New printer technology introduced in 2015 produces high quality objects in minutes. A two–fold change in delivery time happened in only a few years.

The question is not whether we should use surgical robots, but how we can let underdeveloped regions access their benefits. It is not whether patients should measure their vital signs at home, but making sure that doing so doesn't lead to wrong self–diagnosis and harmful self–treatment. It is not whether patients should be able to access their records and medical data, but how to implement and safeguard that access.

In the past we have asked whether to use a certain technology or not. Today we ask how not to overutilize them and still make them accessible to everyone. Ethical issues lie ahead of us, but so do unbelievable advantages. And yet no government, organization, or authority has been able to prepare populations for that. Nonetheless, revolutionary technologies are coming, and we must prepare.

New technologies are increasingly becoming part of everyday life. You can now record health data or check your lab results with a smartphone. You can talk to your doctor via webcam. You can know what illnesses to be aware of based on an online analysis of your DNA.

Hundreds of research trends and thousands of real–life examples demonstrate how reality is getting closer to the science fiction depicted in movies. Supercomputers analyze medical records and draw personalized conclusions. They model how the brain works. Microrobots swim in bodily fluids and might perform small operations soon. External robots draw blood from individuals without the need for human interaction. And yet still I lose days from work when I catch a common cold.

For thousands of years physicians have been the pilots in the cockpit while the patient hadn't even arrived at the airport not having access to their data and the measurements of their body. Now patients are settling into the cockpit due to the swarm of health trackers, but they are not welcome by their physicians. This is the status quo we need to change by putting them there together in an equal partnership. Together they can make better informed decisions.

We are at a stage in which the gap between healthcare technology's potential and what we have in reality has become huge. The only way for human evolution to adjust to the pace of technological change is to embrace disruptive innovations. We need to do so in our jobs as well our healthcare. While robots and the algorithms behind them improve at an increasingly faster pace, we should strive as human beings to improve ourselves and utilize the mind's utmost creativity. If we cannot make this happen, then we will lose the battle sooner than most skepticists thought.

The changes I propose are not going to happen over our shoulders. Only we, individually, can accomplish that. By upgrading our health to a level not yet seen, and improving the skills that make humans extraordinary we have a chance to retain what's really important to us while still improving healthcare worldwide.

From Skepticism To Transhumanism

There are those who are against technology in principle, modern day Luddities. But I will provide examples in upcoming chapters that show why the use of technology will help us retain the human element in healthcare.

Some people fear losing their jobs to automation. For example, the first hotel entirely staffed by androids opened in July, 2015 in Japan. Porter service, room cleaning, and front desk amenities are all done by robots. There is currently a robot that can clean 70% of bacteria from a hospital room in 10 minutes using ultraviolet light. IBM's supercomputer, Watson, can analyze over 1,000 data points per second per patient. These machines take no breaks, or demand better benefits and wages. No human can compete with that.

Ray Kurzweil, the famous futurist and Google's director of engineering, started a movement called the Technological Singularity. As he explained in *How to Create a Mind* and *The Singularity is Near*, technology is advancing at an exponential rate, and there will come a point after which we will not be able to understand subsequent developments. Kurzweil calls that point the singularity because it is similar to black holes from which no light can escape. After the singularity, Kurzeil says, we won't understand what is happening around us anymore.

A related movement, transhumanism, believes the prime goals of society should be improving medicine, health, and technology. It is unethical to die, transhumanists say, and so we must strive for immortality by dedicating efforts to ageing research, genomics, and biotechnology. The popularity of this movement is apparent in the plan for the first transhumanist Presidential candidate, Zoltan Istvan, to run for US President in the 2016 elections.

According to Kurzweil, the singularity will take place, probably in the 2040s, no matter what we do. The event can even be desirable if we take precautions. Transhumanists tend to overemphasize the importance of technology in issues such as creating an artificial womb, cryopreservation after death, or extending life spans to the extreme. Both these movements make points that are applicable to medicine. But I believe that the final answer lies in balance rather than extreme ends of the scale.

We can achieve that balance by using increasingly more disruptive technologies so the human touch can remain at the center of medical practice. The human touch might even be improved. People in underdeveloped regions currently struggle to get access to basic equipment and medical supplies. To them new inventions might look like elements of a science fiction movie that they one day might be able to afford. One way to achieve this is having Internet access that leads to crowdfunding a disruptive medical idea that reduces costs. Other steps forward might be 3D printers that produce inexpensive equipment, delivery by drones delivering to otherwise unreachable locations, machines that print out drugs on site and on demand, and smartphone accessories that measure relatively straightforward health data.

Think of the physician who needs to input a huge amount of patient data every day using traditional keyboards. Or think of the patient who can undergo an expensive MRI scan but pays, travels and waits a lot to get medical attention for even a simple ailment. To change this, a society more interested in and demanding more from medical innovations is needed.

Personalized Healthcare Depends On The Person

People say that applying more technology to medicine will render it faceless. But I think that truly disruptive innovations will lead to customized care as we have never experienced it before. Personalized medicine means that one gets treatment based on one's unique genetic–molecular–metabolic constitution. Personalized medicine may appear to be more expensive than conventional medicine today, but it is cost–effective in the long run because of less frequent hospitalization and fewer side effects. Personalized medicine won't be passive so that we can neglect to take care of ourselves. Rather, it will give us the necessary tools and information to maintain a healthy lifestyle or successfully manage a disease.

The security behind these information tools and the thin line between machine and human present ethical challenges. Instead of ignoring them, we must prepare for their arrival. If we do, then personalized healthcare will emerge individual by individual. It will involve how we live our lives, and what we demand from ourselves, our caregivers, and our governments. It starts with a simple step: try to live a healthy life. If you need motivation, you can find it through your social circles or through devices that act as your personal coach.

In the 1950s, people gathered in homes that had a television, and watched the same program on one of three channels. Now we don't watch TV on TV anymore. We watch on touchscreen devices at a time convenient to us. We used to listen to fixed radio channels. Now anyone can create their own playlists on iTunes or Spotify. In the 1990s, search engines were designed to suggest websites in response to search query terms. Now Google is so personalized that we get different results for the exact same search query depending on our location, what habits we have, or what device we are using.

It seems every service and activity around us has become personalized except for the most important one: healthcare. Identical pharmaceuticals are manufactured for millions of people as if everyone were alike. Guidelines are set for populations rather than individuals. The one service that should be entirely customized is actually not.

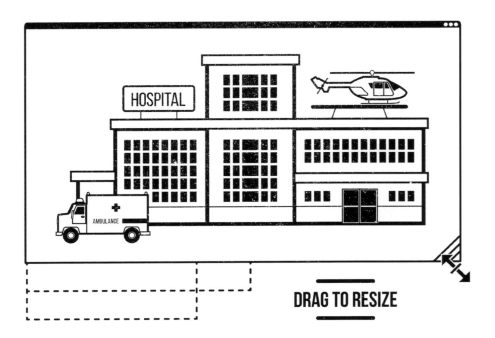

DRAG TO RESIZE

Healthcare worldwide provides mass care in varying quality depending on the finances of the patient or their country. Policy makers and governments might find a way to make care personalized, but we cannot sit around and wait for it to happen. Care will only become customized if we make it so. It has become obvious in the past decades that smoking causes several types of cancer, and that obesity has serious consequences. Still not everyone is fighting against them. If we cannot live a healthy life alone then why not use technology to help us?

There is no need to be a physician to become an expert about one's physical, mental, and emotional health. Favoring technology helps, but by itself it is not enough. To make informed decisions we need to make medicine as personalized as possible by obtaining data that we couldn't previously obtain. I have always wanted to live a healthy life, improve my skills, daily habits, and, more importantly, the way I work every day. Since 1997 I have used both analog and digital methods to help me, and I am still at it. Let me summarize how and then show you the details in Part III.

Analyzing My Own Health

When I was a teenager I got fed up with the mood swings that every teenager suffers. One day you can happily focus on what's important, the other day you are downbeat without any reason. As a pretty rational person I decided to change that. But I needed data to do so. I started assigning a score between one and ten to my daily emotional, physical, and mental state in order to track changes over time. I thought it might reduce my mood swings. It worked. And I still log my ratings every day. Since July 21, 1997, I have not missed a single day. Early on I used simple notes. Now I save my data in a Google document. It takes me seconds a day. This way I can adjust my lifestyle whenever I look at the graph of scores.

I found that my physical score is generally stable and high (meaning good) during the weekdays, my mental score declines over the weekend, and my emotional score is highest on Friday and Saturday. I further found a strong correlation between more exercise and mental performance. As a result I exercise every day so I can focus. Such a simple thing led to important consequences. The data helped me decide what to add or remove from my routine. It helped me live differently and find the balance that so many people are looking for.

In addition to these scores, I have also created a digital log rather than a conventional diary to log what projects I work on, the times I wake up and go to bed, and what I do and think about that day. I have found what things make me sleep poorly, such as certain foods and evening exercise, or what activities result in a low emotional score. I wanted to make my self–improvement as rational as possible – a normal approach for a geek who loves technology and data. For those who don't, it's not much work. I didn't realize I was quantifying myself in reality until about 2010. The wearable revolution introduced a range of devices to my home. My arsenal grew beyond scores and spreadsheets.

I started measuring daily physical activity such as the number of steps I took, calories burnt, or the distance covered with a FitBit I wear on my belt. I use the same device to rate my sleep quality, such as how long it takes to fall asleep and how much time I spend in deep sleep. I saw that it doesn't matter how much sleep I get beyond five hours if I have at least one lengthy deep–sleep period. What I needed to do was simple: find out what choices of drinking, eating, and exercise before bedtime led to a longer period of deep sleep. Now I know. I only need to measure sleep only once in a while now to make sure I'm still on track.

My Pebble smartwatch wakes me with a gentle vibration when I am no longer in deep sleep. It knows when this is because it measures my movements during the night and finds the best time slot when I'm still asleep but in one of the lighter stages. It feels as if I have two assistants, a tracker and a smartwatch, whose only job is to make me have a good night's sleep.

I also measure pulse rate and oxygen saturation (the percentage of oxygen in my blood) during and after running sessions with another device called Withings Pulse. It is literally at my fingertip. If I don't want to be exhausted after a running session, then the Wahoo chest strip that measures my pulse while running lets me know when to slow down. It feels like a personal coach.

A few times a week, I meditate with the Muse headband that measures electrical activity of the brain via seven sensors and transforms them into digestible data. On a smartphone app I listen to the sound of the wind, which the app makes proportional to my brain activity. The less wind I hear, the more relaxed I am. If I can maintain this state for a while, then I start to hear bird song which is the ultimate reward for staying calm. This is how I discovered I hadn't been meditating well for years. The first time I wore the headband during meditation, it suggested that I was far from calm. After some practice I have developed my own method for relaxing myself.

Another small device called Pip that I hold between the thumb and index fingers measures skin conductivity. It provides me with an indirect measure of my stress level. While holding it I have to change a winter scene on a smartphone app to springtime simply by relaxing myself for a set amount of time. The longer I can keep my stress low, the faster the scene changes. The task takes me about 15 minutes, while my wife does it in about 4 minutes. Of course it stresses me to think about how much more stressed I am than my wife, at least according to the device. But I am working on it.

Every vital sign is at my fingertips. A smart blood pressure monitor from Withings that I have provides a visual diagram of my readings. I use an AliveCor ECG bracket on my smartphone to record my electrocardiogram. The app gives me a basic analysis of whether there are any abnormalities. If I need a professional reading of my electrocardiogram I can get it within hours for a reasonably small price, or I can send it directly to my general practitioner in PDF format.

I can improve my attention by piloting the Puzzlebox Orbit drone using another headband studded with sensors. If I focus long enough, I can launch and then control the drone through my smartphone. This is not really safe to do at home, but it is quite spectacular. I don't use these devices every day, and certainly they do not control my life. I do. But for the first time I can pilot my own health by the use of such new innovations.

From Devices To Online Services

In addition to devices, anyone can order blood analyses or genetic tests from home. I learned, for instance, what mutations I carry and what drugs I am sensitive to. A company sent me a tube in which to provide a sample of saliva. I sent it back. In return I got an analysis of the DNA in my sample cells. I learned whether I had a higher or lower risk for certain conditions compared to the general population. For example, I changed my lifestyle on learning that I have a mutation that increases blood clotting, and thus my chance for thrombosis, eight times higher compared to the general population. I also found out that I'm unusually sensitive to caffeine and metabolize it faster than others. Knowing this has helped me shape the way I live and, hopefully, improve and prolong my life.

I had the bacteria living in my digestive tract tested. A company called uBiome performed genetic tests on my microbiome, the population of microorganisms that live in my gut. The results suggested changes I might make to my lifestyle and diet.

I enjoy playing games on Lumosity to improve my mental flexibility, attention, and memory. I listen to music backed by research on Focusatwill. com to focus my attention for long hours when I need to. This kind of classical, jazzy or up tempo music has been shown to generate focused attention for sustained times. The company shared the results of an experiment in a white paper about such music initiating greater organized firing of nerve cells. In other words, neural synchronization increased.

Medical services can take place online today. Smartphones can send high–quality photos of skin lesions to a Swedish company called iDoc24, which analyzes them and provides medical advice through its app, although they warn that the service cannot substitute for a physician visit. American Well, Curely, Healthtap, and hundreds of other companies provide video and text conversations with physicians situated worldwide. The patient uploads medical records and basic symptoms, and then the physician engages in a short phone call, videocall, or e–mail discussion. The fee is paid online. Patients who lack access to a physician turn to these kinds of online sources, as do those who seek a second opinion. I remain confident that even better resources are yet to come for anyone with an Internet connection.

Services, devices, and wearables that provide clinical quality data are changing the way we look at healthcare delivery. Personally, I bring my smartphone to my primary care doctor. We can focus on pressing issues instead of spending time measuring my blood pressure, for instance, with an old analogue device. I am not yet my general practitioner's favorite patient, but this approach is what physicians should expect to see soon everywhere. My doctor is coming to realize that it's easier to work with my kind. Technological changes in general make me optimistic about the future of medicine even though at the moment that future isn't as bright as it might be.

Most patients are not ready for such changes. Many medical professionals are not open to them. It is an entirely new situation for everyone in which the old hierarchy of medicine and the rapid development of technology are colliding with one another. It should not be a fight, and it doesn't have to be.

Ideally, what should evolve is a secure and well–tested protocol that introduces disruptive innovations in everyday healthcare, ones that are affordable, comfortable, and efficient while still being evidence–based. Right now we are at stage zero. The way technology will truly change medicine hasn't even revealed itself yet. But change is coming soon.

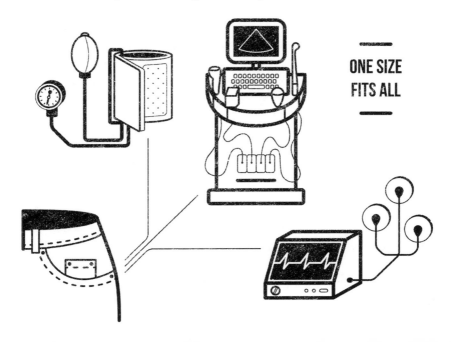

ONE SIZE
FITS ALL

Science Fiction Is Not Fiction Anymore

As a science fiction fan I have watched movies from 1927's *Metropolis* to masterpieces of recent decades. *2001: A Space Odyssey, Alien, Avatar, Inception, Blade Runner, Star Wars*, and similar movies have all depicted future technology that might become real one day. That day has arrived.

After watching *Blade Runner*, I became worried about replicants from the future. In 2001, it was hard to side with either the humans or the machines in *A.I:. Artificial Intelligence*. In 2015, I had to resist the temptation to fall for the lead robot in *Ex Machina*. Cinema shows us some struggles and obstacles we may soon have to face and the possible directions we may go.

The 1966 television series *Star Trek* featured a medical tricorder that gave instant read–outs after briefly scanning a patient. It was a small, hand–held device unlike anything available back on Earth at the time. In 2015, the Nokia Sensing X Challenge solicited engineering teams to design prototypes in the spirit of the fictional Star Trek tricorder. The prototypes will have to measure a range of biomarkers using only a small dropplet of blood. They might monitor epilepsy, diagnose malaria, or intervene in a variety of conditions.

The Alien prequel *Prometheus* featured a surgical robot that performs operations entirely without human assistance. The lead character got injured, entered and closed the doors of the surgical chamber, and then had the robot perform the operation. At present, sophisticated surgical robots are quickly forcing surgeons to develop new skills that are closer to playing video games than wielding a scalpel. At certain universities in the US, medical students are being taught to use gaming devices, which in turn are used to train future surgeons.

The 1997 film *Gattaca* depicted the dark side of genomics. It showed a society in which genetic differences and even predispositions make some people superior to others. As services that provide genetic data become easily accessible to laypersons; governments and organizations are working to defending people from discrimination based on their genetic disposition. *Gattaca*, whose title comes from the four nucleotides of DNA – G, T, A, and C – is a dystopian example of why an individual's genetic information should not be public or shared with employers and insurers.

In the futuristic world depicted in *Elysium (2013)*, a mother put her daughter into a machine that looked like an MRI scan. It diagnosed acute limphoblastic leukaemia, a cancer of blood cells, and simultaneously cured her in seconds. In the film, not everyone had access to the machine, which led to rebellion. In our world, radiology equipment is constantly getting smaller, more comfortable, and smarter. Portable ultrasound machines can be attached to a smartphone, and the physician can transmit the image to a specialist who can check it out. At the Fraunhofer Institute for Medical Image Computing in Germany hospital surgeons use a tablet device coupled with the radiology images in order to zoom into the organs before opening patients up. *House, MD* would have loved to have looked through patients that way in the TV series. Now it is possible.

In the 1997 movie *The Fifth Element*, a fragment of DNA found in a hand allows the characters to print out flesh, bones, and nerves in 3D in seconds. The result was a living human being. As of 2015, it has been possible to print out tissues such as blood vessels, bone, heart valves, ear cartilage, synthetic skin, and even functioning liver tissue.

In *Robot & Frank (2012)* an elderly patient is given an android, a human–like robot, by his son. The son intends it to be a companion with artificial intelligence that can do shopping, clean up the house, and converse about everyday issues with its owner, Frank. The robot subsequently becomes a real friend. Today, Honda's humanoid robot, Asimo, can take the stairs or motivate people to exercise more by dancing with them. Asimo has more than 50 degrees of freedom of movement which means it can move its body in a lot of ways in three dimensional space. The NAO robot has even more, and impressively has performed the famous Evolution of Dance, a viral video from the early days of YouTube. Such robots will soon be commonly used in homes of the elderly and in emergency situations, saving people's lives.

In the movie *Her*, released in 2013, an artificial intelligence operating system replied to and organized hundreds of unread e–mails for its user in a second. It kept track of every task and appointment of the main character who started to have feelings for the cognitive computer and its voice. No surprise given that Scarlett Johansson was that voice. To what extent could we improve our lives if we had such a smart companion? To what extent will the cognitive computers currently working with physicians improve patient care?

Hacking the human brain has likewise been a topic of recent films. In *Lucy (2014)*, smart drugs significantly expand the capabilities of the human brain. This leads to unexpected and dramatic consequences. *Inception (2010)* showed how we might plant an idea into someone's subconscious. Actual brain implants currently help people with epilepsy or Parkinson's disease. Retinal implants give hope to individuals rendered blind by a genetic eye condition, retinitis pigmentosa. Such implants have been approved by the US Food and Drug Administration (FDA).

BBC aired a documentary series called *The Real History of Science Fiction*. It told how creators of science fiction movies always have to think ahead and look beyond. They must create things that other scientists are too conservative to imagine. Sci–fi screenwriters and directors are bold by nature, which is why we eagerly await new releases. In them we spot technologies that could change our lives in the near future. For decades, innovators, inventors, and medical companies have stolen ideas from Hollywood. It's time to move medical technology forward so quickly that Hollywood will have to steal from us.

Watching and reading science fiction has never been more useful for preparing us for the coming waves of change. I urge you to watch as many movies and read as many books as possible. They will introduce you to ethical issues we have not yet encountered but surely will. Science fiction can change the way we look at medicine but it doesn't necessarily improve it. The gap between what it depicts and what patients experience is growing. This creates an awful feeling when people see amazing developments but rarely get access to them.

Once people get a clearer picture about which innovations might improve their health, they are going to demand it. Why, they ask insurers, isn't my prosthetic device cheaper with 3D printers? Why, they ask their physician, can't I get the most advanced targeted therapy in cancer? Today's society must make sure that financial disparities do not lead to biological ones. Being more charming, smarter, faster, or taller only because one can afford it should not be an issue.

Why Don't I Get The Robotic Arm From That Movie?

One force behind the growing gap between fiction and reality is financial. Most people living in countries that have either private insurance or socialized medicine cannot afford the latest state–of–the–art health technologies. No healthcare improvement or economic policy will be able to truly change this. Only revolutionary technologies that deliver better, less expensive, and more efficient care can make those wheels turn.

3D printing, for example, decreases the cost of prosthetics and exoskeletons. Distant care services don't require people to travel for hours for a lab result or miss days from work. Comfortable wearable devices could measure vital signs with the same quality as more expensive equipment does. Rapid technological advances finally give us a chance to make care affordable to people worldwide. The optimism of that last sentence stems from one simple innovation that was introduced in 1991: the Internet.

With an Internet connection you can crowdsource whatever information you need from any experts by using social media channels. Dave deBronkart, leader of the e–patient movement, has tens of thousands of followers on Twitter and Facebook, and even more readers on his blog. Dr. Kevin Pho, a leading physician voice in social media, has hundreds of thousands daily followers. Social media channels from Twitter to Pinterest and Instagram give medical professionals, patients, and organizations an opportunity to have their voices heard and get answers to specific questions.

Salvatore Iaconesi, a programmer in Italy, discovered that he had brain cancer. Taking the initiative he gathered his medical records and scans from hospitals. But he received them in different formats. His programming skills let him create a digital repository in which to analyze all pieces of information. He posted this on a website, La Cura, meaning "The treatment" in English, in order to gather insights from people around the world. Such an opportunity is currently the privilege of those with digital skills and those who speak English. But this will change.

You can 3D print a prototype of an idea without having to pay manufacturing expenses. 3D printing services are becoming available worldwide. Even large stores have them. Typically, one creates a virtual model with 3D software or a scanner, and then the printer produces it in a few hours. A new method introduced in 2015 reduced the hours–long process to minutes. That is an example of a disruptive technology. Improving a feature by making it ten, a hundred or a thousand times faster and cheaper.

If you need financial backing, you can crowdfund an idea without having to knock on doors of investors. People can back a project with a commitment: if the project raises enough money, they will pay the amount they specified. The Star Citizen video game raised $74 million. A portable cooler raised $13 million, and the Pebble Time smartwatch raised over $20 million in a month to finance production. Now some companies use crowdfunding as a test to see whether there are enough people interested in buying the product. Small startups can get the initial funding for transforming their idea into reality. The only thing matters is if the idea is good enough.

As Peter Diamandis described in his book *Abundance*, billions of people have never been online and their ideas are still yet to get discovered. The coming years will see the democratization of ideas. Being original and disruptive is going to be more important than whether the idea comes from the Silicon Valley or Central Africa. Credentials and country of origin will matter less and less, while the originality of an idea will persuade increasing numbers of people to risk their money and time to make it happen.

You can see for yourself by checking how the editorial system behind Wikipedia works. It doesn't matter where you come from or what degrees you have. If you provide good references and quality information, you're in. Major journals such as Nature or The Economist have encouraged the research community to follow blogs that express opinions and points of view you will never find in peer–reviewed papers. Democratization sounds great in other industries and can happen relatively easily. But in medicine, where hierarchy has a thousand years long history, it is going to be difficult if not dangerous.

There is a reason why it takes not years but decades to become a competent medical professional, and no online service or home monitoring device can match that. At the same time patients should take more responsibility for their health. Achieving that is not so simple when many people have lost faith in numerous applications of modern medicine.

Losing Faith In Modern Medicine

Healthcare systems in underdeveloped regions – if you can even call it a system – face problems different from those in developed nations. Institutions worldwide contend with the lack of latex gloves or basic equipment, not with the absence of 3D printers or state–of–the–art radiology devices. In developed regions, physicians get burnt out easily dealing with information overload, administrative headaches, and having to see a greater number of patients in less time than before.

Improving healthcare is not a matter of money. Healthcare spendings in the US compared to its GDP is the highest in the world. Yet the US is not among the top 30 countries in average lifespan. „The more we spend, the better it gets" is not true any longer. I once read an amusing article about what restaurant bills would look like if they operated like hospitals in the US. They would charge for greeting the diner, taking an order, or even letting you sit next to the window. The soap in the toilet, the stove usage would all have its price; similarly to the waiter delivering the bill or the cashier making change.

Worldwide, 142,000 patients lose their lives because of preventable events such as inaccurate diagnosis, treatment, injury, or hospital–acquired infection. Certain medical errors have fortunately resulted in reformed delivery of care. For example, fetal heart monitoring during labor lets physicians intervene if needed; using markers to avoid amputating the wrong limb; counting the number of sponges used during surgery so that nothing is left inside the patient. Today medical records, treatment plans, health parameters, and much else is digitized–and yet the number of medical errors is still growing. These contribute to about one fifth of annual deaths in the US. The capitalistic nature of developed countries' healthcare systems doesn't help to rectify this.

The key performance indicator for a hospital is still its financial figures and not the actual success rates of doctors. No system can be improved and maintain a level of quality without measuring its elements all the time. Like a pilot that has all relevant data on a dashboard, hospital managers should be able to steer an institute to better performance. They should be able to fill in niche areas, or redirect hospital–based physicians to activities they have time for at the moment. Doing so could eliminate hours of waiting time for patients. With chronic conditions, this might add up to weeks of waiting time. With big data at hand, solving inefficiency would no longer be rocket science.

Such efficient systems will need medical professionals who can deal with data and new technologies, and who are ready to adjust to a new status quo. They will need to orient their patients to the digital world and act as role models of healthy living. This is certainly not the case right now. I have been teaching medical students how to acquire skills that help them become better physicians in a technological world. Becoming better means offering empathy and truly listening to their patients.

An efficient system will also factor in the unrealistic demands of patients who have seen the latest technology on television or in film and demand that they get them. Yet there will be caregivers who cannot answer questions related to the digital world. Meanwhile, empowered patients will get rejected for being up–to–date, and this will disencourage them. The system we call medicine has been around for over two thousand years. There are physicians who are still educated to make decisions for their patients and wield more parental responsibility than they should. Similarly, there are patients who are socialized to be passive and think that „The doctor will tell me what to do." And there are technologies that already started changing this just a few years ago. Naturally it causes trouble. Sometimes chaos. But it is going to get much worse unless we upgrade our skills and health.

Financial problems, unrealistic demands, and physician burn–out all contribute to a loss of faith in modern medicine. In 2012, 33% of US adults used some form of complementary medicine. Fish oil was No. 1 according to the National Center for Complementary and Integrative Health of the US. Dr. Ben Goldacre, a physician, journalist, and author of *Bad Science* has debunked alternative medicine, poorly conducted research, and unethical practices by health "gurus". Recent peer–reviewed studies have concluded that alternative medicine does not work. And yet its popularity remains stable. One possible reason for this might have to do with not needing health insurance or expensive referrals to access it.

The communication skills of those working in alternative medicine are crucial. They can persuade the patient to choose unsound alternative methods over proven medical ones. Their success might have to do with their emphasis on the one key element in the caregiver–patient relationship: attention. This is something modern medicine does not do well anymore, or does only in private, expensive settings such as concierge medicine.

Good technology can change that. With better devices and algorithms, doing jobs that physicians cannot do, doctors could be relieved to focus wholly on the patient. This optimistic view is not without grounds.

The Success Story Of Modern Medicine

Modern medicine is full of success stories. We have successfully eradicated smallpox, and global eradication is underway for poliomyelitis, malaria, measles, rubella, and many more infectious diseases that have killed millions of people. The world average of life expectancy at birth increased from 47 in the 1960s to almost 70 in 2015. It is projected to go past 70 by the 2040s. By that time it will be more than 80 in the most developed regions. That is a lifespan increase of almost 40 years in just decades. Surgical planning, anesthaesia, in vitro fertilization, early cancer detection, and fetal ultrasound are among the best examples.

Physicians could restore the sight of someone blind for decades by using his own stem cells. Patients born with limb deformities or those who lose them in accidents could get robotic prosthetics they control with their thoughts. Ever–improving therapies in AIDS, and gene therapies targeting genetic mutations or cancerous cells are becoming more widely available. Common chronic conditions such as high blood pressure and diabetes can be well managed with new medications and approaches. Modern medicine has significantly changed our lives compared to earlier decades, and unrecognizably so compared to people in the 19th century and earlier.

Still, most people fail to recognize this amazing rate of development because good is never enough when it comes to one's health. We expect diagnoses to be immediate and perfect. All treatments should be without side effects or complications. Cancer should be merely a bump over our lifetime instead of being a dramatic event. We are never going to get cured passively with one pill. Our contribution is needed and this is the essence of care.

Interactions that patients have with the healthcare systems are only part of the issue. A much larger chunk is self–care, which ironically is and has always been the main form of medicine. Given modern advances one might get the impression that self–care will play an increasingly smaller role. But failing to take care of ourselves before calling on our physician might be the biggest threat to the future of medicine.

This should be where all begin. For example, I take care of myself by becoming expert at reading my physical, emotional, and mental health. When I need help, I turn to an expert caregiver. As this notion of becoming the experts of our own health hasn't improved over the last decades, we can assume no change will happen. But with better technologies, motivation can increase as they make health quantifiable outside the hospital settings. It has not been possible before. And as technology went forward, it became accessible only to those within the healthcare system. Again, not anymore.

Wearable devices, smart clothes, and medical equipment have already changed how we live. In a matter of years, smartphones, tablets, and smartwatches have become common sights. I can access major vital signs and track changes via smartphone applications. Small attachments can do things like measure blood alcohol, diagnose malaria from a drop of blood, or detect ear infections. Such possibilities are becoming widely accessible to anyone inside or outside healthcare.

The genetic backgrounds, or genomes, of thousands of people are currently available. The cost of sequencing one person's genome was $3 billion in 2001. It is roughly around $1–2,000 in 2015. The cost keeps on decreasing. The genetic data are used to prescribe personalized drugs in customized dosages. Doing this avoids unnecessary hospital readmissions and adverse side effects. In certain types of cancer, such as lung or breast cancer, targeted chemotherapies to which the tumor cells are sensitive are already being used. And yet we are still nowhere compared to where these opportunities will bring us in the coming years. We cannot expect physicians to lead this new movement.

They already deal with information–administrative–patient overload. Ironically, policy makers and governments have never known less about upcoming changes than they do now at a time when they should be the most up–to–date. We cannot change systems without changing the approach of the people in them. Patients, for example, have never been allowed or encouraged to disrupt healthcare, even though they could be the main hackers of care. It is obvious that things have to change. And there is one major driving force that will make it happen.

Breaking Down The Ivory Tower

For thousands of years medical information and even devices that measured vital signs have been accessible solely within the ivory tower of medicine. Only trained professionals could learn methods, secrets of care, and access information in peer–reviewed studies. While the hierarchical and patriarchal structure of medicine has remained essentially the same, the surrounding world has changed dramatically in the last few decades.

Starting in 1991 the Internet has taken over everything we do – from buying groceries to keeping in touch with friends. First the mobile phone and then the smartphone put this digital jungle into our palms wherever we go. As of 2015 Facebook had over 1.3 billion users. More messages are sent via Whatsapp than by text messaging. Websites such as WebMD and MedLinePlus give health information to millions of users who search online every day. Medical studies have become available to anyone via Pubmed.com, a database of biomedical studies. Everything has changed, except medicine.

Fortunately, the rise of the empowered patients who are informed, get the information they need, bring it to their caregiver, and wish to take part in making decisions about their lives has started to break down the ivory tower. Empowered patients know how to use social media and the digital jungle. They are up–to–date about their condition. They ask for second opinions. They get advice from fellow patients who are going through the same issues. Happily this saves time and effort for them and their caregivers, making the ivory tower no more. Anyone can access more than 23 million medical papers on Pubmed.com. They can measure almost any kind of health parameter. Yet it seems that time is needed for people to adjust to the loss of the ivory tower.

Physicians need to leave it and meet patients half–way. This step alone disrupts a thousand years–old industry, and I'd like to dissect the thought for a moment. Physicians are fundamentally trained to become god–like figures to patients who tell them what to do, what therapy to follow, and what drugs to take. No one ever argued against this before. Students had to study for a decade before becoming physicians, and then practiced for decades more to accumulate as much clinical expertise as possible. They learned to use medical equipment and communicate their findings. This model has lasted for hundreds of years. Check out the television series *The Knick* directed by Steven Soderbergh for a more detailed insight into the early days of medicine to see what struggles practitioners had to endure to provide today's quality of care.

I have heard many stories in which patients tried to read up about their condition online only to have physicians get angry and try to maintain their authority over decision-making. Physicians who resist empowered patients are not keeping themselves up–to–date. If they did, and if they followed the literature closely, they would know that involving patients in the decision process correlates with higher satisfaction.

When I was a medical student in mid 2000s being left with a clinical problem I had never before faced made me feel awful. I wanted to feel connected to a network of medical professionals. A few years later social media turned out to be the solution. For more than a decade I have enjoyed the advantages of being connected to tens of thousands of like–minded professionals by selecting them one by one and getting help whenever I need it. Every medical professional and every empowered patient should be allowed to feel connected to many others who can help professionally or emotionally when they have questions or just need a good word or support. Social media can become this bridge people need.

The Ruins Of The Ivory Tower

It is simple to create a new status quo once the ivory tower breaks, although its implementation takes time. Both medical students and practicing physicians have to acquire new skills like digital literacy worldwide, not only at certain institutions. Instead of being keyholders to the ivory tower gates, they can be the patient guides in the digital jungle. This is a huge transition. Resistant physicians will face mounting difficulties in dealing with such patients, or they will have no job at all. They need to learn new technologies and be able to choose the most suitable ones for their work. This may be devastating given that the medical profession is known not to embrace change. The coming e–patient tsunami will, however, disrupt that.

E–patients will quantify themselves and take health application data to their physician because they want to make decisions jointly. Doing so will force their doctor to become better at this integration, or otherwise they will align themselves with somebody else. This happens to be the main driving force that shapes healthcare in the developed world.

If, with proper education, we can bring physicians down from the ivory tower and make their job better, save them time, and prevent burnt–out, then patients also need to take an important step. They need to embrace health management. The vast majority of patients only start caring about their health when they are sick and receive a diagnosis. This diagnosis is usually a major life event because up until then they hadn't had to focus on their emotional or physical health. After the diagnosis often come unrealistic demands of getting cured with a pill without having to change one's lifestyle. This scenario is simply not going to happen.

Patients instead need to take care of their own physical, emotional, and mental health. Smoking, excess alcohol, and bad diet can no longer be elements in a normal lifestyle. To accomplish this we need to make a healthy life rather than fitness attractive and trendy. This challenge is bigger than that of transforming physician approaches. Fortunately for patients it is becoming easier to live a healthy life than not to. Technology can now quantify how healthy we are and how we might improve it. We have to grab the chance and make people proactive so that they take health matters into their own hands.

Patients who are experts about their own health and physicians who are experts in their profession can together make the best decisions. It might sound overly optimistic, but it isn't. Patients should sit in the driver's seat, but the car should be automated. By that I mean that patients should control what happens to them. They should own their medical data. But what the patient goes through while receiving care should depend neither on human error or luck. It should be well–designed and automated by smart algorithms and similar technologies. Where is the physician's place in this analogy? Sitting next to the patient.

Roles Have Always Been Changing

Moving closer to the technological revolution changes roles in healthcare. Patients become empowered and proactive. Physicians get better at using digital solutions. Policy makers become informed about what is happening in technology, and discussions become initiated on the public level. Such role changes have not yet started in our technological era, but new inventions have sped up the process.

Researchers use entirely different methods than they used to. Instead of recording observations and drawing conclusions, instead of seeking information in libraries and writing down discoveries on paper, they now work with huge databases covering biotechnology to economics and use supercomputers to analyze them. They disseminate research findings on scientific social networks such as ResearchGate. Findings appear in open access journals such as PloS.

Nurses once wore uniforms, oxford lace–up shoes, and distinctive caps. Decades ago patients stayed in hospital longer (11 days compared to 4 now, on average). Typewriters and glass thermometers were once common. The only way to lift a patient out of bed was by a strong nurse. Nurses today provide a growing percentage of primary and chronic care. They routinely access information about pharmaceuticals and physical procedures. Automated beds, cieling–mounted lifts, and even robots have become somewhat regular. Nursing has become increasingly specialized job and one condusted in partnership with physicians.

But every role in healthcare has been changing. So why would the medical profession and the most important player, the patient, not change?

There once was a time when touching the patient –the laying on of hands– was not a part of the physician's visit. As a result uroscopy became standard: visually examining the patient's urine in a bottle for symptoms of a disease. Practitioners of the time could diagnose diabetes, jaundice, inflammation, and even tumor by looking at the temperature, color and other features of urine.

Much later medicine divided into specialties. Physicians became scholars to find the reason behind certain medical conditions. Autopsy became a common element in medical education. Herman Boerhaave, a Dutch physician, introduced bedside teaching in the early 18th century because he wanted to reinforce theoretical knowledge with first–hand bedside observation. His new method traveled through Europe and transformed medical education.

Not all developments are futuristic. Up until 1816, physicians listened to heart and lung sounds by putting their ear against the patient's chest. This embarrassed female patients, and it was impossible to hear much if the patient was overweight. René Laennec, a French professor of medicine, invented his stethoscope after seeing children play with long, hollow sticks. They held their ear to one end of the stick, which amplified the sound if the opposite end were scratched with a pin. Observing this, Laennec designed his first instrument as a 25 by 2.5 cm hollow wooden cylinder.

He presented this invention at a meeting in 1818, but the medical society failed to embrace it. Even the founder of the American Heart Association at the end of the 19th century carried a silk handkerchief to place on the wall of the chest for ear auscultation. Laennec died from tuberculosis at the age of 45. His instrument was developed further by others to reach the standard it has today.

Portable ultrasound let physicians actually see what so far they had only been listening to. Dr. Eric Topol states in *The Patient Will See You Now* that he hasn't used a stethoscope in years given that he can see the heart via portable ultrasound. Changing technology constantly shapes the way physicians do their job, but the last years' innovations have pushed this truism to another level. Technology is now too fast to comply with current regulations and laws.

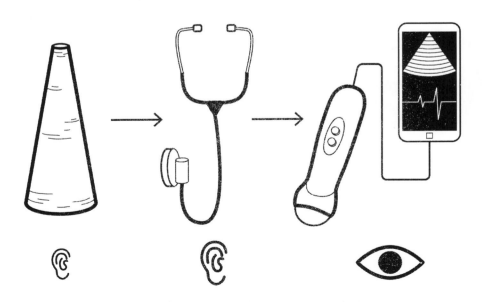

The 20th century brought lab markers and blood tests to everyday medicine. Medical education became mass production after World War II. Physician disengagement from patients started to accelerate even though insurance made healthcare available to many more besides the rich. This disengagement expanded the gap between patient and physician, and between technological advances and everyday medicine.

The role physicians play today will not be the final role they will play in healthcare. It will keep improving. The last few decades have demanded much more from physicians than they could humanly deliver. They should be up–to–date, have a scientific approach to medicine, empathize with and pay attention to patients, collaborate, publish, educate students, learn new technologies, and improve constantly even as administration, regulations, and legal threats of malpractice get worse.

No physician can gather all knowledge about a field of interest or specialty. Nor can he acquire sufficient experience and communication skills to convey their thoughts to patients perfectly. Patients should share some of this responsibility not only because it concerns their own health, but also because it would liberate physicians to do what they are best at: dealing with patients. This will not happen without using more and more technological applications.

Imagine cognitive computers that gather all necessary information. Devices that let physicians move around their data as they would in their minds. Gadgets that measure important health parameters, freeing up physicians to listen to patients and talk with them. These are simple examples. But to implement futuristic technologies in everyday healthcare, we must be able to see where we are heading.

Can We See What Is Coming Next?

In 1995, I received an AMIGA computer that I fell in love with. Since then each computer I've had has had more and more computing power. In the 1990s my father had one of the first mobile phones. It was the size of a suitcase. Smartphones and tablets surpassed PCs in 2014, and the real story is just about to begin. As a geek I grew up with keyboards and thick monitors. Touchscreens only got into my life in my 20s.

Kids can so intuitively search for cartoons on YouTube now that existing technologies have become boring before they even get to primary school. Amazingly huge networks of devices and people who share every moment of their days will be major components of their lives. If they do not develop skills that make them at performing certain tasks better than robots or algorithms, then they will have no job at all.

If Baby Boomers born between 1946 – 1964 and Generation X born between the 1960s and 1980s think they are challenged by technology, then the Millennials and Generation Z will continuously face such challenges during their lives. It can be a good thing if they are prepared to adjust. Certain philosophies and movements champion this direction.

The technological singularity predicts serious consequences for humanity from the technological explosion. Artificial intelligence may well develop its own superintelligence and control a swarm of nanorobots that can basically do anything it wants. Cosmologist Stephen Hawking and Tesla founder Elon Musk both expressed their fear about how artificial intelligence might destroy humanity. James Barrat described methods we could use to stop or at least slow this process. Nick Bostrom, expert of artificial intelligence, explained potential scenarios that superintelligence might lead to.

Dr. Eric Topol has been a leading voice in digital health, advocating for the use of smartphones and patient empowerment made possible by technology. Others simultaneously caution the excessive use of technology given that it removes the human touch. With such battling forces it has never been harder to get a clear picture of what is actually happening in medicine.

Instead of trying to predict what comes next, what if we looked only at the most promising directions? Doing so requires exponential thinking and the ability to look for trends in other industries. Here is why.

In Paris, French artists designed a series of post cards for the 1900 World Exhibition. Their goal was to depict the year 2000. They made plenty of strange predictions about how education, transportation, households, music, and our daily activity would change. Perhaps they were limited by linear thinking, and missed the point of exponentially developing technology around them.

They thought, for example, that robotic orchestras would perform in music halls. But then why not digital music? Creating digital music is far simpler than teaching robots how to play the violin. They thought we could transmit knowledge to the minds of students simply by putting books into a machine and turning the handle. We can transmit thoughts through electrodes but don't have digital data? We really need to digest printed books for that? The list of examples could go on for about 80 post cards.

Linear thinking is „a process of thought following known cycles or step–by–step progression where a response to a step must be elicited before another step is taken". Technology no longer follows this step–by–step rule. We have to adjust our approach to the future to account for that. I am not saying that every technology has accelerated at an exponential rate, but they have certainly gone beyond the linear stage.

A second example concerns a young architect in North Korea who got a chance to envision the future of North Korean cities. He came up with ideas for a green metropolis. In one drawing the interior design had a rotary dial phone on the bedside table. Like those architects who had limited access to modern ideas, if we cannot look outside our own field, it will be impossible to make useful predictions.

Linear thinking and the inability to look outside our own field will prevent us from seeing key trends that shape the future. We need to be brave when dreaming. For example, the Kaiser Foundation sponsored a facility in the 1950s: the hospital of the future. The patient's record reached the doctor through pneumatic tubes before he reached the patient. The hospital featured big lights in the operating rooms. Mothers could check their newborn babies in a sliding drawer. Although some of these elements have become common in hospitals today, others fortunately have not. If we do not dream big, then important steps toward improving medicine will take decades rather than months.

Small steps are no longer sufficient. We need technology that is revolutionary, less costly, more efficient, and more secure than anything that has come before.

Good Technologies Disrupt Industries

Two things are certain given the past decade's changes in medical practice. Technology itself will not solve the problems that healthcare faces globally. If it did, then better technology would immediately lead to better care, and that has rarely been the case. But the human touch alone is no longer enough. Many physicians and patients think either technological advances or the human touch will rule the future of medicine. But I think that both will.

The time during which a patient meets his caregiver in person is a sacred one. It is a privilege relatively few people enjoy. So how about making it a common commodity of healthcare?

In other industries, inaccuracies or imbalanced developments of technology; as well as the lack of regulations regarding brand new methods might cause problems; but in medicine it is going to cause chaos. Healthcare is a generally sensitive industry with a lot of limitations, strict rules and the one thing everyone is concerned about, their health.

If it doesn't deliver the same quality, results and steps forward other industries can due to new technologies, people will turn away from it looking for alternative solutions. This is a scenario only snake oil salesmen look forward to. The cost and availability of delivering care will not decrease dramatically under current circumstances. The only way to make care affordable is including disruptive innovations that can not only change the system but entirely disrupt it.

Car manufacturers have been improving cars since the early years of the 20th century. Nevada was the first US state to pass a law permitting the operation of autonomous cars. In 2014 Google unveiled a 100% autonomous car without a steering wheel or gas pedal. It had logged over a million kilometers. The car cannot yet recognize policemen or temporary traffic signals, and it has had only minor accidents as of 2015. Google hopes to make it commercially available by 2017. If all goes according to plans, it will revolutionize transportation. Fewer cars will be on the road, traffic flow will be better, parking will not be an issue, and we will be able to work while traveling. Imagine the hours added to our regular week by such an invention.

Elon Musk, founder of Tesla, thinks of his company as an automobile and software company. The software in Tesla models is constantly being refined even when the driver is sleeping at night. New models can navigate in the dark thanks to sophisticated sensors, but the technology is currently ahead of legal regulations. The company is in contact with US regulators about when these new capabilities might be officially activated in vehicles. Countries such as Germany are developing the infrastructure for charging electric cars on motorways ahead of companies, and encouraging the use of electricity instead of carbon fuels. Over time electric cars could render cities colder due to their decreased emission of carbon dioxide.

After the television boom in the 1960s came VHS cassettes in the 1980s and 1990s. After that CDs, DVDs, and then Blue–Rays became the standard formats for watching movies. In the 2010s, online streams revolutionized not only how we watch TV, but even how series and movies are made. Netflix spent almost $500 million for producing new shows in 2015. And yet still many countries have no clear regulations whether such streaming services can be legally used or not.

Amazon made a big announcement in 2014 that it would soon deliver products to a buyer's doorstep by drones within minutes after placing an order online. The US Federal Aviation Administration then gave permission to use aerial vehicles as prototypes for delivery. Unfortunately those rules became obsolete during the process of issuing the regulations.

Uber is becoming a global transportation company that allows consumers to submit a trip request to crowdsourced taxi drivers. It democratized transportation by taxi even though critics in many countries say it is unsafe and illegal to use unlicensed drivers. Still, they raised over $2.8 billion in funding, and Uber is available in over 50 countries and 200 cities. The process of using this business model has become known as Uberification.

Google acquired startups or companies involved with deep learning, artificial intelligence, and robotics. A company in the latter category is Boston Dynamics that has a real menagerie of robotic animals and humanoid robots such as Petman. Google broadened its knowledge and experience in robotics more by buying out a dozen companies in the past two years than any other company or institution had before. It also began collaborating with Johnson & Johnson to design surgical robots.

Nestlé, the food and beverage company, opened a division for 3D printing food. We don't 3D print food at home, and only a handful of companies are focusing on that possibility. But Nestlé saw opportunities in the field and wanted to be prepared by the time it becomes a common practice in the home.

Cosmetics giant L'Oréal started working together with Organovo, the US company that prints out liver tissues that can function like a biological liver. L'Oréal's intent is to produce synthetic skin to test their products without limitations. A food company that wants us print out food at home and a cosmetics company bent on producing synthetic skin sounds like science fiction. But it is happening now.

Many large companies realize the potential of various technologies and try to anticipate in what directions they might be headed. Failing to act now might put them out of business later. Similar foresight is needed in healthcare. If we don't act now, technology will take over and be autonomous. No one wants that to happen.

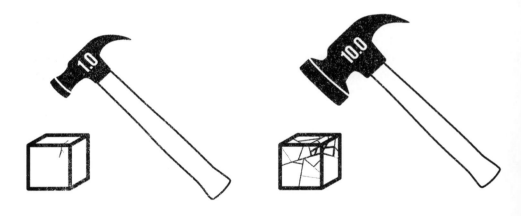

It Is Time To Upgrade Our Health

Human biology has its own natural upgrade cycle. In other primates the brain stops growing at birth. The human brain continues to produce new neurons until about 2 years of age, and the brain is not fully mature until about age 25. In barely two decades we undergo hormonal and metabolic metamorphoses. In the immune system new antibodies form to fight microorganisms. Elsewhere molecular changes lead to or prevent diseases. After age 35 we start losing thousands of brain cells daily. Women stop ovulating in their fifties. All this is to say that a lot of biological changes already happen in the body without the need for our interaction. Nonetheless, we can influence some of these processes by gathering data about them, making lifestyle changes, or bringing about direct molecular changes through technology.

Typically, software gets upgraded, people don't. By upgrading our health I mean incorporating technology into our lives in a way that it improves health or mitigates disease. Upgrading in this sense means using more technology to gather data; make good decisions; and improve general well-being as a consequence. The term might sound as if my intention is to emphasize technology over our biology, but I mean just the opposite. Our health can be improved, and the humanistic element of medical practice enhanced through the embrace of disruptive innovations. In fact, I think this is only going to be possible by using technology even more than we use it already. If we want to upgrade health globally, then disruptive technologies must be available in all regions and to those with any financial background. If this isn't possible, then the technology is not yet good enough.

It took the telephone 75 years to reach 50 millions users. The same audience took radio only 38 years to build, 13 years for television, 4 years for the Internet, 3.5 for Facebook, and only 35 days for the smartphone app Angry Birds. Medical innovations will not reach that many people as quickly. Barriers include regulations which are strict for a reason. People also tend to care more about communicating and smartphone apps than their own health. Technology applied to medical practice strikes many as removing the human touch.

Doctor shortages throughout the world cause serious gaps in providing even basic care. The World Health Organization estimates that there is a worldwide shortage of around 4.3 million physicians, nurses, and allied health workers. No medical curriculum will be able to solve that within the next decade. Yet ethically, care must be provided. Remote care or "telemedicine" has been tried with some success. The rapid appearance of new technologies recently may make this a reality in more parts of the world.

Digital stethoscopes, wearable devices, ECG smartphone brackets could measure all the vital signs and health parameters. Robotic telecare devices could deliver the physician's face and sound in great quality. Usually only the handshake and the physical examination are missing. Force feedback gloves that let users touch objects and let others feel the same from a distance wearing the same gloves have been around for some time and they should significantly improve in size and quality in the coming years. Then, the handshake and even the laying on of hands would be possible.

Someone not getting care because of a physician shortage could finally get medical attention. Some would object that it goes against the traditional structure of medicine because it takes place in different geographical locations. Such critics like to think that people can only provide care the way it has been done for thousands of years. Greek and Roman civilizations' healers diagnosed and tried to cure people with tools such as forceps, scalpel handles, hooks, and spoons.

Later physicians found cures without the need for superstition, but with a focus on the scientific method. The 20th century was about further improving that method which became evidence–based medicine in the 1990s. When hospitals started doing more systematic analyses of patient symptoms with respect to diagnosis, the volume of data became too huge to humanly analyze to say nothing about keeping up with it.

We can acknowledge the limitations of the human mind and turn for relief to tools we have created. Cognitive computers, augmented reality, 3D printing, and genomics all have the potential to disrupt healthcare. And dozens of similar technologies will do that immediately except we are not ready for that to happen. We cannot learn the details of every new innovation, and it shouldn't be our job. What we can do is to start searching for our own motivation for change.

My wife goes out for a run because I go with her. I go out because I can measure data using wearable devices. It doesn't matter what kind of motivation helps individuals stay healthy or improve their jobs. What matters is that a person finds that motivation himself. No organization or government will ever change healthcare from the top to the bottom. Only we can do that individually by being proactive.

We need to live up to the expectations of living healthily, upgrade our health with better technologies that maintain quality of care and keep the human touch. We can become familiar with technological developments, learn the ethical issues, and initiate change ourselves. Waiting lists and issues of affordability, and accessibility can be resolved with revolutionary technologies that are already available. We are in this together.

Let's start by changing the way we take care of ourselves and continue to improve those things we are good at. Such a market will generate bigger demand from companies; thus inventors will drive development. The next years present a tipping point in human evolution, as well as a once in a lifetime opportunity. Let's not miss it.

I am optimistic about medicine's future because current trends all seem to point there. Medicine will become more patient–centric, more efficient, and more digital. And yet empathy and sensitivity will be as central as ever. Patients will become more mindful of their emotional, mental, and physical well–being. They will want to be partners in their healthcare with physicians who will have the time, energy, and focus to interact the way patients want them to.

Many technological developments will make this possible. Policy makers will be able to look at big data and draw the best conclusions for how to reshape healthcare delivery. Poorer regions will access basic care with telemedicine, 3D printers, and that one Internet connection. Health is going to be a prime social issue regardless of philosophies or movements.

As I began to examine real–life examples of the technological revolution and their possible influence on medicine, I became increasingly enthusiastic about the advantages, but simultaneously concerned about threats and ethical issues. In the next chapters, I present both positive and negative sides in order to get a balanced picture about where we are and where I think we should be heading.

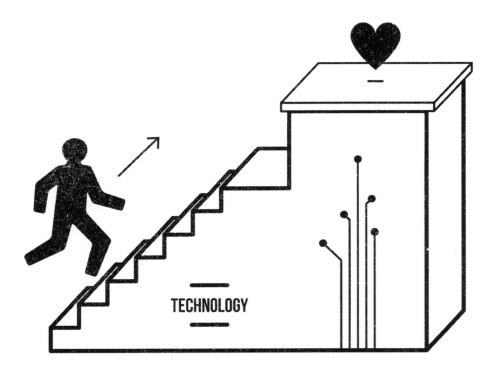

PART II. THE MOST EXCITING QUESTIONS ABOUT THE FUTURE OF MEDICINE

Because no current medical system is ready for a coming technological explosion, ethical issues will increase in the coming years. We must also address bioterrorism, controlling medical devices from a distance, financial differences that lead to biological ones, privacy, and transhumanism. It will help to initiate conversations at home, at work, and in the public sphere. We need to understand what is coming to be able to deal with the waves of change, and to upgrade our health.

Start by asking how our lives will change. How do we want them to? How much will we allow technology to transform the way we live? How dangerous will it be if we do not prepare society for breakthroughs? Discuss these questions with experts and laypeople. It is a wonderful first step.

I have been having such conversations for years. I give a lot of talks every year, flying from event to event to discuss the need for public deliberations on the pros and cons of technology's effect on medicine. While I like to speak as a medical futurist, the questions that audiences ask are often fascinating and cover a surprising range of issues. Medical professionals, industry experts, young entrepreneurs, students, and patients have asked me more than a thousand questions over the last decade.

Students ask mostly about how they can prepare for coming changes. Physicians ask whether they will be replaced by robots. Industry experts ask about business opportunities. Engineers ask about practical solutions, and how devices might be better used in the home. Patients tend to ask about ethical issues and what they should do for their own medical condition. Patients ask me questions they already asked their doctors but didn't get satisfactory answers to.

Some of the patients sounded optimistic, others curious. Yet others were angry or worried about the future. I enjoy being challenged, and I have been challenged many times. Sometimes these questioners came up with ideas that transformed the way I look at the future. I'm grateful to them for this.

A few years ago I started making notes of the best of these questions. My note taking was not only about questions but also the story behind the persons asking it. There had to be a reason they were worried, skeptical, enthusiastic, or angry. I had to realize some answers might be evident to experts working in digital health, but not for laypeople who are at the same time more affected by the answers.

I felt moved to share the answers with those who could not attend a particular conference or get the answers they wanted from an authority.

The next chapters highlight the forty most exciting and interesting questions I have ever received. The answers are meant to clarify every topic, ethical issue, and potential advantage. Given that Twitter is probably the most mainstream channel for such discussions, I use #hashtags that can help locate others who are also interested in the particular materials. As a movie buff I also cannot let you miss the relevant movies. These you will find under each heading.

I divide questions into three groups. "Everyday life" contains answers that affect the way we live, eat, or work now. "Disruptive Trends" presents the most promising directions and technologies, from 3D printing to artificial intelligence. "And Beyond" suggests the wild future of society, and things we cannot see yet. I invite you to discover how technology could, will, and shouldn't transform our lives.

CHAPTER 1. EVERYDAY LIFE

WHY WOULD YOU MEASURE YOUR ECG AT HOME?

#wearables #digitalhealth #mhealth | Robot & Frank (2012)

In the first days of the so–called wearable health revolution, which resulted in an arsenal of devices monitoring health at home, I gave a talk in London about how I had been quantifying my health for decades. I described how I gave scores to my mental, emotional, and physical well–being. And then how I started measuring my vital signs, sleep quality, and daily activities to improve how I live. I also demonstrated some of the gadgets I use. Afterwards a physician stood up looking a bit angry and asked me in a really sarcastic tone why I would measure ECG at home. He seemed offended by the possibility that patients might measure such parameters behind his back.

This is a typical reaction. Certain physicians feel that they might get left out of the picture if patients access things that they could only access through their doctor before. I'm working hard to prove them wrong. I assume this particular questioner meant that there is no need for patients to measure every health parameter, and that there is a risk of over–use of such medical devices without proper supervision. He would be right. But this question raises bigger issues than he might have imagined. My initial answer to him was simple. I measure because I can. I see no reason for doing an ECG regularly at home. A friend of mine who is also a physician told me jokingly that if her husband had this opportunity, he would do an ECG every five minutes.

Having the chance to measure whatever I want to measure feels great. Now that more devices are becoming commercially available (and who knows how many others are on the verge), it's hard to clearly see how to use them appropriately. This (r)evolution started at the end of the 2000s with a few trackers that could measure the number of steps a user took each day, the distance they covered, and maybe how many calories they burned. In the early 2010s people started measuring other things from body temperature and sleep quality to brain activity and even feeding time for babies.

A 2014 report showed that 71% of 16 to 24 year–olds want wearable technology. Industry predicts a 2018 market value of $12 billion, and shipments of 112 million units. One–third of Americans will own at least a pedometer.

Google's Fit and Apple's Healthkit made steps forward but still cannot fill the gap between data measured and what comes next. If you have those apps on your smartphone, they will measure the number of steps taken, distance covered, and calories burned. Other apps and devices can be added to your phone so that it aggregates your data into one system. It is far from being the personal coach we might like to have, and it will unfortunately also eat up your battery time.

The ECG device I mention in my talk is AliveCor. I hold a small device to the back of my smartphone and it immediately starts showing my ECG on the screen. After 30 seconds, it analyzes the data and reports any abnormalities such as atrial fibrillation. Atrial fibrillation is a leading cause of stroke that can be prevented 75% of the time if detected and treated in time. I can also request professional advice from ECG experts who will remotely interpret it within hours for a small price.

The company's founder, Dr. David Albert, told me it had hundreds of examples of people who recorded irregular heart rhythms and e-mailed the ECG to their physician. Some people with palpitations have been told by their physicians that it was only anxiety. AliveCor has shown that these people sometimes have serious heart problems. Over fifteen peer-reviewed papers on different clinical applications together with case studies from leading heart centers such as Cleveland Clinic show that this is not a gadget, but rather a medical device that people happen to be able to buy over the counter. One study pointed out that patient feedback regarding the ease of use of such a device was also positive.

Measuring a health parameter is empowering. Checking myself no longer makes me totally dependent on the healthcare system. Over-use, making inaccurate assumptions based on the data they provide, or not having accurate measurements are all major problems, but I still believe freedom is more essential. Members of the Quantified Self movement have been promoting this since the 1970s when the first very early wearable computers became available. Members measure whatever they need to address problems, whether it is bad sleep or losing weight. They also work in groups where they share what they learned and how they changed a habit or lifestyle. Quantified Self has gone from fringe to mainstream.

If you cannot decide which wearable to choose, Lumoid, a company known for its short-term camera rental service, offers a wearable package containing five different health trackers that users can try before buying. After deciding, you send the package back and purchase the device directly from Lumoid's online store or through other vendors.

A DIY wearable movement has also sprung up. People who can code can create their own personalized wearable device. It contains GPS, measures whatever they want to measure, and the design depends only on their imagination. As coding knowledge becomes more common, the gap between the makers and the users of technology will close. Consumers will start to look at devices and services in a different light. They might change their behavior and thus the way companies develop new products.

Chris Dancy became famous as the "most connected man" on Earth. With a ton of gadgets and sensors he made his home smart. If it senses Dancy losing his temper, it pipes Classical music into the rooms. Dancy looks at qualitative data in the form of surveys he sends to himself. For example, he analyzes his heart rate and brain activity with activity trackers and a head-band that detects EEG. Doing so has enhanced his contemplative practice in ways he never expected and has helped him deal with his panic attacks and depression. He began to see correlations elsewhere. For example, his caloric intake increased when he watched several episodes of the same TV show. He realized that he eats better when he sleeps more soundly, and that he sleeps better if the air quality is better. Making changes was easy.

Dancy sees three forces driving this kind of shift in personal health management. First, people can find anything in the world but nothing about themselves online. And yet they want to understand their life. Second, a class of physicians and allied providers is emerging that understands how to use data measured by patients that will personalize services. Third, all devices, services, applications, and sensors from Facebook to FitBit are currently using or will soon use our biological behavior to drive what experience we have while using them. Our behavior is about to become a track pad and our life a programmable experience. Ethical issues related to that will be the new "privacy" debate.

Dr. Danny Sands, a primary care physician in the US and –authority on digital health has no argument with patients wanting to know more about their bodies. But a fundamental problem is that more information is not always better. If it were then we would order total– body MRIs, multi–panel blood chemistries, and full genome analyses on everyone. Human biology is not an engineering problem in which if we only had enough data we could diagnose and treat everything. Whether devices are accurate or not, and variability from person to person are valid concerns. So is provoking needless anxiety by positive findings that don't mean anything and for which no action is necessary. Or worse, false positive results lead to unnecessary and possibly harmful interventions.

The more we do, the more likely we are to find something. There is a high likelihood that things we "find" lead to treatments that are risky, expensive, and do not improve life at all. Dr. Sands urges patients to collaborate with their physicians, but he also believes that office visits are not needed unless absolutely necessary. Follow–up, especially for chronic conditions, can be done from home without necessitating a visit if an illness remains well controlled.

This is the kind of meaningful use we should work hard to achieve. The devices behind this movement are still in their infancy. Some devices are not sufficiently accurate, do not provide useful data, or promise too much. There is no reason to believe there won't be improvements in the coming years. Although just started, the revolution already is playing a role in breaking down the ivory tower. What happens when it's gone depends on us.

Reporters and curious people have experimented with wearable devices. Many concluded that they did not help them make lifestyle changes. I'm certain that the above adopters did not get the most out of them. Perhaps they even used them in the wrong way. A device is just a tool that gives me something I couldn't access any other ways. Or maybe I could get it only in the hospital or in my doctor's office. What the wearable trend brings is freedom. It gives patients a chance to become experts in themselves.

I don't measure ECG on a regular basis at home, nor should anyone else without a medical reason. But having the chance to do so whenever I want is liberating. Likewise I do not measure my sleep quality every night, and I don't carry my Fitbit with me every day. But when I do I enjoy making informed decisions based on what the devices show because I can. Having a technology break once in a while and going to bed without any gadgets on me help find and keep the balance.

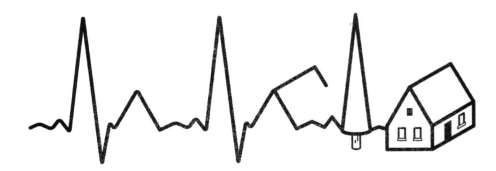

WILL TECHNOLOGY CHANGE THE LIVES OF PEOPLE WITH DIABETES?

#diabetes #wearabletech #dsma #dayofdiabetes
Steel Magnolias (1989) Memento (2000)

I give talks organized by patient associations or public events that are attended principally by patients. I like talking about what digital channels they could use to manage their illnesses. What social networks would help them find others coping with the same problems? I also like to talk about how technological revolutions will affect them. I hope to motivate them to become pilots of their own health by sharing real-life stories with them.

At a 2015 meeting in Central Europe I discussed what technological breakthroughs were expected in the months ahead that could help manage several conditions. Given that diabetes is a major target of such efforts I was not surprised by the first question, which was posed by a woman who was also a mother. She wanted to know if technology could change the lives of diabetics. Both of her daughters had the disease.

It is of course wrong to offer false hope by promoting advances that are not yet available. I have to be careful with the wording, but being an optimist I cannot hide my excitement about promising developments. Diabetes affects 400 million people worldwide. It can benefit greatly from new developments in sensors, big data analysis, and online services. Here are a few examples.

Amazing applications for smartphones can help manage diabetes efficiently. MySugr, an Austrian company, released a set of applications that add gaming to traditional diabetes apps. Gaming aims to motivate patients so that they get their blood sugar under better control. The app imports values from the patients' blood glucose measuring device, enters the values into a logbook, and has a Quiz feature to improve understanding of diabetes. MySugr Junior is a companion app for kids. It teaches them how to manage their diabetes by taming a little monster. Kids earn points for every entry they make, and the goal of the game is to score a particular number of points on a regular basis. It also lets parents keep an eye on the results remotely.

VoyageMD aids diabetics who need to travel. It provides up–to–date information on traveling with diabetes, including reviews of places to stay, travel itineraries, checklists; travel product reviews, and tips for airport procedures.

Devices and apps generate an awful lot of data. A website called Databetes offers a digital way for logging and measuring meals and their effect on blood glucose. It also came up with the novel idea of analyzing the big data behind one person's disease. The idea came from founder Doug Kanter who tracked all his diabetes data for an entire year with activity trackers, food logs, glucose meters, and a number of apps. As a result he improved his lab markers, lost weight, and achieved the best control of his blood sugar he ever had.

In addition to accumulating data, patients also need support from one another. Social media has become the best channel for that. Individuals can coach each other. Kerri Morrone Sparling is a prominent example of how someone can become a leading voice in the diabetes community by sharing her experience and opinions on a blog at Sixuntilme.com. Connecting online and in person reassures people living with diabetes that they are not alone.

Social media has saved lives in her diabetes community. It has helped those who struggle to improve control. It shows people that there isn't such a thing as a "perfect diabetic," but there can be an educated and determined one. It doesn't encourage people to wallow or become resigned. Instead it serves to inspire them to do the best they can, and to seek out the best healthcare they can find at home and in the doctor's office. A strong support system makes a tremendous difference for someone living with diabetes.

When it comes to pocket–sized gadgets, MyDario designed a smart meter that plugs into a smartphone. It includes test strips, a lancing device, and completes its measurement in 6 seconds. Abbott pharmaceuticals released the FreeStyle Libre system in 2014. A water–resistant wearable sensor takes glucose readings with a painless one second scan that can be transmitted wirelessly to the smartphone even through clothing.

A similar skin sensor can measure glucose levels by using an electric current to draw glucose to the surface. In a few years it will seem barbaric that diabetics once had to monitor their blood sugar by pricking themselves and releasing a droplet of blood onto a single–use test strip.

Most people have heard of Google Glass, an augmented reality device. Google has also patented another augmented reality device in the form of a digitally–enabled contact lens. An ancillary feature is that it calculates blood glucose levels from the sugar content in tears. Google has formed a partnership with the pharmaceutical company Novartis to develop smart contact lenses that can track diabetes and also correct farsightedness.

Food scanners are an invention that can count exactly how many carbohydrates a given meal contains. TellSpec, a Canadian company, plans to release such a food scanner in 2015 that additionally will determine how many and what kind of ingredients, allergens, toxins, carbohydrates, or calories a food actually contains. Diabetics can then base their meals not on best guesses but on concrete data.

Insulin pumps infuse insulin under the skin as an alternative to multiple daily injections and doses calculated according to blood glucose monitoring and carb counting. A better approach is to monitor blood glucose levels continuously and base the pump's dosage of insulin and glucagon accordingly. This will be directed by a computer algorithm that mimics how a healthy pancreas does the job. This would in essence be an artificial pancreas, a closed-loop insulin delivery system. Engineers from Boston University have already developed such a bionic pancreas. They plan to begin clinical trials in 2016.

Diabetic complications necessitate an amputation every 20 seconds worldwide. In the US more than half of these amputations lead to death within five years. These grim statistics led researchers to invent Smart Sox. These intelligent textiles are made not entirely with thread but contain fiber optics and sensors. It was developed to identify motions that are problematic which could serve as an early warning sign of diabetes complications.

Two other exciting technologies are on the horizon. The first is smart insulin that activates in the bloodstream when the blood sugar exceeds a preset level. It then switches off when sugar levels return to a normal range. The second development is encapsulation therapy. This prevents the autoimmune destruction of insulin-producing beta cells in the pancreas. Many diabetics doubt that a biological cure will happen in their lifetimes, but these kinds of promising technologies offer hope and optimism.

Diabetes is only one example of a disease that has profound and widespread consequences. The management of many conditions from Alzheimer's to heart disease will dramatically change soon. There is, for example, a smart spoon for Parkinson's disease patients called Lift Ware that adapts to their hand tremors so that patients can feed themselves again. Technology can help people manage diabetes and other conditions in a gamified and comfortable way.

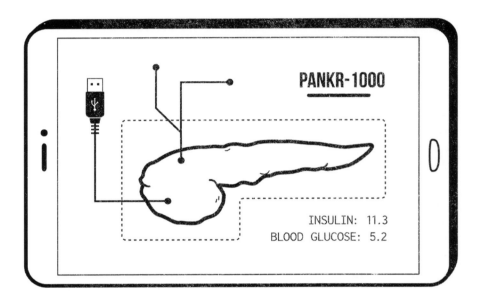

WILL PEOPLE MEASURE VITAL SIGNS AT HOME?

#wearables #digitalhealth #QS | Big Hero 6 (2014)

A multinational insurance company contacted me. They wanted to address the wearables' revolution before their competitors did. They invited me to give a motivational talk. The CEO asked for my most counterintuitive examples because she wanted the sales staff to see what the future of healthcare might hold. I did as she asked. When I was finished a country manager stood up, looked skeptical, and asked whether people would measure their vital signs at home. From his tone it was clear that he thought they would not even though trends and statistics showed him to be wrong.

Living a healthy life is harder than not doing so. It takes effort, time, and frequently costs more. But a healthy lifestyle should be considered a long–term investment into ourselves. Being able to function better for longer will be its own reward. Finding daily motivation is a struggle. People with self–discipline can maintain their motivation. Others need help and incentives of different kinds.

First, one has to change behavior. Anyone who has tried to lose weight, quit smoking, or put down a smartphone knows how hard breaking habits and adopting new ones is. Some people must try multiple times before they succeed. Others get discouraged early on and give up. Changing behavior without having data and clear rewards is almost impossible. Groups such as the Quantified Self and Weight Watchers have been collecting and analyzing data about its members for decades. Not until the 2000s did we have devices that made data collection easier and more comfortable. The wearable revolution brought the means of breaking habits into our homes.

The Tinké device measures cardiac fitness and lets users compare their results to different populations. FitBit sends me weekly updates about my activity level compared to the previous week. Withings notifies me when I reach a new goal such as walking 1000 kilometers. Muse persuades me to engage in relaxation sessions by showing me how many points I need to keep my average every week. Scores, points, badges and other elements of gamification might be a solution for people who want to change specific behaviors.

In one clever experiment in Sweden, piano keys replaced the stairs at a metro station. When people stepped on them they generated sound. The experiment asked what percentage of commuters would choose the stairs instead of the escalator or elevator. Amazingly, 66% of them did. After all, people like to play. If we keep this in mind we might persuade them to exercise more and live a healthier life all together.

According to BJ Fogg who leads Stanford's Persuasive Technology Lab, we need three conditions for a desired behavioral change: having access to essential resources such as time and money, being motivated and receiving triggers while changing a habit. If one of these is missing then the change is unlikely to happen. If one or more conditions are in place, all that is needed is providing the missing condition. Smartphone apps or devices can do this.

I spoke with Jurriaan van Rijswijk, Chairman of the Games for Health Europe Foundation, about why it is so hard to adopt new habits. A gamification expert, van Rijswijk, says that motivation is one factor in changing behavior, but loyalty towards the subject of change is something people usually don't consider. The money versus time issue is often why desired long–term behavioral change fails. He gave me a practical example.

Take the common example of wanting to exercise more. We start buying gym clothes, a pair of new shoes or a mountain bike. At first we are enthusiastic. But gradually we exercise less and less, and spending increasingly less time at it makes us less committed to our goal behavior.

If, instead, we first started spending time exercising with limited resources and technology, such as using a smartphone app to motivate us and provide rewards that trigger a desire to exercise, then gradually the new behavior becomes valuable, and we will spend our valuable time doing it. Once the perceived value of exercise gets higher, we will happily spend money in order to spend more time exercising.

The key to success is time commitment or loyalty to the subject. Technology is a resource liberating tool that helps us spend more time on the desired goal. The best interface for that is a game. A game works as an automatic collector of vital signs. It can act as a buddy to keep people motivated and give them triggers at a pace and frequency that reinforces the desired change in behavior.

Designing games for this is complicated, but there are good examples of apps and services that provide motivation and rewards, and reinforce commitment. There are those who are not motivated by a device or their credit card being charged with a monthly gym membership. Their bike might be in the garage ready for action and still they don't use it. They need to constantly look for new solutions because there must be at least one type of motivation that will work for them. Everyone can be motivated with the right methods. It might be an app, a device, a runner buddy or making the process fun for ourselves.

Mango Health developed a smartphone application designed to motivate patients to take their medications on time. Users set the times when medications should be taken, and the app reminds them. It also provides information about the medications, and warns about drug interactions and side effects. By taking the medications properly, users earn points towards gift cards or charitable donations in raffles held weekly.

WellTok created a platform, CaféWell, which engages consumers by getting to know them and building a Personal Health Itinerary. It is a personalized action plan based on their interests, health status, activity level, and other demographics. It initiates small, achievable acts, and recommends digital resources to help users achieve large improvements over time. It also rewards them along the way.

Blue Shield California, a not–for–profit health insurer, attempts to make wellness fun via social media. Participants earn points, badges, status, and see their progress. Blue Shield claims that 80% of its employees have participated, and had a 50% drop in smoking prevalence.

The Didget blood glucose meter, which connects to a Nintendo DS gaming platform, is intended for kids between 4 to 14. It helps manage their diabetes by rewarding them for consistent blood glucose testing. As points accumulate, new game levels and options unlock. There are leader boards with kids who collected the most points, web games and an online community as well.

EveryMove collects data from trackers and apps we already use to allow friends to compare one another's progress. Social motivation, such as seeing that my friends went for a run today but I haven't yet, is a strong one.

Insurance companies in increasing numbers have decided to build on gaming by adding incentives to their health plans. Fortune magazine named Oscar the "Hipster health insurance company". It hopes to become the Spotify or Uber of health insurers. It offers subscribers a wide range of physician services, keeps track of their medications, logs important events in their care, and uses tech–based incentives. Members receive a free Misfit Flash fitness tracker they can synchronize with the Oscar application. They earn $1 whenever they hit their daily goal. The reward can be $240 each year just for being physically active. Fortune noted that some people were concerned about sharing their data with an insurance company, and that is a risk decision makers have to address. Imagine eating a big sandwich with a lot of red meat, and your tracker reporting the number of calories to your insurance company, which then increases your rate based on this bit of data. We wouldn't like insurance companies to play such a "Big Brother" even if we would like it to reward us for healthy living. Until we become proactive ourselves for the sake of getting healthier, a range of gamified apps, services, and devices is ready to help us become so.

If you don't like gamified solutions off the shelf, you can create your own game. For instance, I assigned scores to my health every day and gave myself rewards if I kept up a healthy habit for a predetermined length of time. Find what will motivate you the most and build on that. It's going to be worth it.

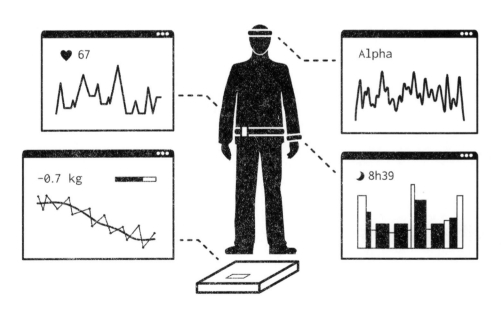

CAN TECHNOLOGY REALLY IMPROVE MY SLEEP QUALITY?

#SleepHealth #wearables | The Machinist (2004) Inception (2010)

I was on my way to a television interview when the taxi driver asked me what my interview would be about. I told him I had been invited to talk about how technology can change healthcare. I described wearable devices and how some of these could improve my general well–being a great deal, especially the quality of my sleep. He became interested because he had been sleeping badly for years. We had time during the ride to tell him how I improved the quality of my sleep step by step (I describe this in Part III).

As he listened he kept asking why he would measure his sleep when he has no idea what to do with the results. This is a problem that stumps many patients. Even if they did start using devices to collect health data, making lifestyle decisions based on it is difficult. We need to be patient. A few years of development has produced dozens of devices that will eventually get smaller, more comfortable, cheaper, and more user friendly. My optimism arises from the observation that wearable devices can provide guidance about lifestyle. They don't have to be perfectly personalized. Trial and error lets patients implement small changes first and see whether they work or not.

Imagine using a sleep tracker that shows you your sleep quality in the morning, including how much time it took to fall asleep and how many deep sleep periods you had. It asks how you feel in the morning. If you are not energized it suggests what to try before the next night. For example, it may say get hydrated, or don't have dinner after 8 p.m. It continues to assess your sleep. If it seems to improve you have just discovered a new approach to ensure a good night's sleep. If it doesn't improve, the device will offer other suggestions crowdsourced from other users' habits. In time you will gain a lot of experience about how to make your sleep quality adequate. Eventually you can use the same method but without any device telling you what to do.

We cannot expect individuals to come up with their own solutions; technology has to develop and help in this direction. Companies are designing devices and services that suggest how to change lifestyle in order to improve sleep or general well–being. For example, the web app Exist.io collects data from whatever apps and services we use for health tracking. It gets data about our e–mails or checks in at places, and it tries to come up with useful tips.

Last night I had the best sleep I'd had in days, therefore, the app suggested, let's do the hardest tasks today. Another time it might tell me that people are more likely to walk when it's colder at night and tonight is going to be cooler than average, so let's take advantage of it.

According to the Sleep Foundation, adults need seven to nine hours of sleep. This works out to spending one–third of our lives asleep. Sleeping five hours or less each night increases mortality from disease or accidents by 15%. Sleep quality is complex. It depends on an individual's genetic background, lifestyle, habits, and factors such as light, humidity, and noise. But why rely on circumstances when we can take steps to have a sound sleep ourselves? It is impossible to maintain emotional well–being, sharp mental activity, and be generally healthy without quality sleep. With the right technology, we can improve it dramatically without much effort.

Withings developed Aura, a device that uses a contact–free sleep sensor tucked under the mattress. It has a bedside light–and–sound device and a smartphone app that were designed to promote sleep onset by maximizing the correlation between light wavelengths and the secretion of melatonin, the hormone associated with the sleep–wake cycle. Its smart wakeup function times itself to the user's personal body clock. It can bring the user up to a light sleep level with special lights shortly before it's time to wake up. Beddit is a similar sensor that users can sleep on top of. It assesses sleep quality via respiration, heart rate, sleep cycles, and sleep duration, and it suggests ways to sleep more soundly.

I only use my tracker when my sleep has been disturbed. I want data to make changes and restore it. As soon as I'm back on track there is no need to use the device. During my exploration phase I tried another device that was strapped to my arm. It made me look like a cyborg, which amused my wife. It measured oxygen saturation and a slew of other parameters, but in the morning it showed me exactly what a poor sleep I had during night. But it was bad because I wore the device not because I did anything wrong before bedtime. This anecdote emphasizes that devices are not the solution: my decision to improve the quality of my sleep is.

More gadgets will appear on the market soon, but they are worthless unless you want to change the way you sleep. Nobody will sleep better because a device tells them to. You need to take the first step by being proactive. Then a device can help you. It should serve as a personal coach that gives you personalized advice. Technology can reinforce lifestyle changes, but the decision to change is always yours.

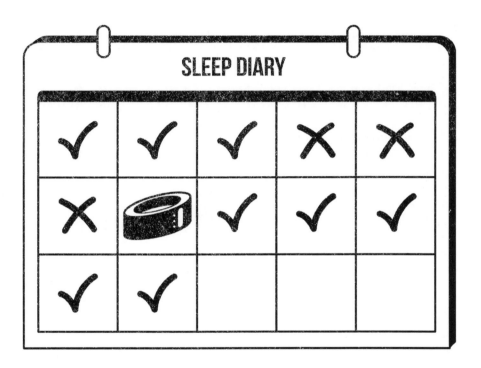

IS IT POSSIBLE TO SCAN FOOD FOR INGREDIENTS?

#foodscanner #nutrition | Star Trek (1966–1969)

I often blog about trends that promise to have the biggest influence on medicine in the coming years because it is hard selecting auspicious technologies out of the hundreds of different developments and it is my job to provide possible directions. These posts receive the most feedback from people around the world. After I published my predictions for 2015, a mother left an emotional comment about her daughter of 8 years–old who was allergic to many foods.

She told how hard it was to find food her daughter can eat. She had to check labels diligently for allergic ingredients, and she had to cook conscientiously. She was pregnant at the time she wrote and was worried. Were there any labeling advances or technological devices that could make her life easier? Was it possible to scan foods for their ingredients?

Extrapolating from European statistics, 220 to 250 million people may suffer from food allergies worldwide. In the US one out of three people has a food allergy or modifies the family diet because of a suspected food allergy in a family member. Approximately 5% of children, and 4% of teens and adults have clinically proven allergic reactions to foods.

Globally, about 35% of adults are overweight, with half a billion being obese with a body mass index of over 30. According to The International Diabetes Federation, around half a billion people will have diabetes by 2035; half of them will be undiagnosed. Food allergies and diabetes are only two examples in which knowing calorie intake and ingredients are pivotal in managing daily medical issues.

Given these statistics, the European Commission launched a prize challenge of €1 million to develop an affordable, mobile, non–invasive solution that enables users to measure and analyze their food intake. The contest runs until the end of 2016. Hundreds of other similar initiatives are needed to help people deal with diabetes or obesity.

We really have no idea what we eat now. We can only guess. Ingredients are listed on most of the products we buy, but every meal and every plate is different. One remedy would be having a list of exactly what ingredients and how many calories a meal contains, and what allergens and toxins might be in it. I mean not just the kind of meal we eat but the actual food on our plate and its specific amount. Several companies have been trying to address this.

The Canadian TellSpec company had a successful crowdfunding campaign in 2013 that raised more than $380,000. Now it aims to develop a hand–held food scanner that can inform users about specific ingredients and macronutrients. Through spectroscopy, an analysis by how matter interacts with different wavelengths of light, it can quickly determine the chemical compounds in a given food. The company founder, Isabel Hoffmann, had a story similar to that of the mother who commented on my blog. Hoffman's daughter got sick after the family moved to a new flat in Toronto. Months later the girl was found to have a variety of food allergies.

As a result Hoffmann recruited a team to design a device that could tell what was in a particular food. That way she and others could know what to avoid. They sent out the first devices to beta testers in mid 2015. Several critics have raised questions about the device and whether the company can deliver what they promised. Some backers in the crowdfunding campaign seem willing to wait and see.

Another device, SCiO, from Israel, was founded by people with optical engineering backgrounds. They have raised over $2.7 million on Kickstarter in 2014. It uses a technology similar to TellSpec's but is designed to identify the molecular content of foods, medicines, and even plants. It illuminates an object; optical sensors detect the reflected light; and the device analyzes it using an algorithm and a cloud–based database that is constantly updated. The company promises that in milliseconds the ingredients and molecular make–up of the foodstuff appears on the user's smartphone. The device was scheduled for shipment in 2015. But many backers lost patience when the deadline passed. On top of that experts in applied science criticized both companies for overstating what their inventions can do.

There are two major issues. One is size, because the device must be hand–held to become popular. With current technology this means something has to be given in, such as sensitivity and accuracy, in order to achieve a convenient size. The other issue is the algorithm. SCiO sends data to the cloud which then sends its calculation back to the device. But to simplify what the algorithm has to do, users need to tell the scanner whether the sample is a solid food, a liquid, or vegetable. This inconvenience is the price one must pay to keep the scanner small.

There aren't any promising hand–held food scanners on the horizon besides these, but there is no reason to believe a solution will not arise in the coming years. The challenge is not when a workable device comes along but what we will do with the large amount of data it generates. Let's say a scanner tells me how many grams of sugar my fruit contains, or what the alcohol percentage of a drink is. So what? It won't change my behavior and dietary habits unless I'm a dietitian, and even then it's far from clear why it would. Perhaps its progress will be similar to that of wearable devices and sleep trackers.

A good food scanner should accurately determine ingredients, and compare the data to my lifestyle, dietary choices, and my genomic background. Given how different we all are genetically, two people might digest the same food at a different pace. One might be allergic to an ingredient while the other is not. So far, pure luck and experience have alerted us to these differences. It should not work like that. Eating should be a conscious process where we know what we eat, and know what we should eat for optimum health. A food scanner with a smartphone application could fill this place.

But let's not leave out an interesting side note here, namely, incorporating genetic information into food scanners. I already have the data of my complete DNA sequence at home in a digital file. Literally thousands of studies speak to the genetic aspects of nutrition, a field called nutrigenomics. I should be able to learn what foods and individual ingredients are bad for me. Genetic tests showed me that I'm sensitive to caffeine and process alcohol more thoroughly than most people (I'm Hungarian after all).

Nutrigenomics tries to understand how nutrition affects our metabolic pathways, and what we can do to get the most out of nutrition in a personalized way. If I choose the other type of meat or cheese as the smartphone app suggests based on my DNA, I will enjoy the meal more and take a better care of my body on the long–term. With access to such data a scanner or app could tell us what products not to buy at the grocery store, what type of food makes us more productive, sleep better, or just feel healthy. Right now we're depending on blind luck.

Wouldn't this be an overly technological world where devices, scanners, and apps tell us what to eat and do? I prefer to look at it from a different angle, from the benefits of finally knowing what we eat and what ingredients lead to positive and negative consequences. I see customization to my specific genetic background as another benefit, too.

Diabetes patients would know how many carbohydrates their food contains. But knowledge doesn't change behavior alone, otherwise nobody would smoke. Knowledge supported by gaming or technologies revealing our lifestyle choices to our family members or caregivers might do.

Patients with rare genetic metabolic disorders such as phenylketonuria would know what to avoid at all cost. Having a good diet would not rely on the experience we bring with us from childhood and what we have learned since then. Instead, it could be based on informed decisions. If it means a food scanner should become a commodity in my life for this, count me in. I want to know what I eat.

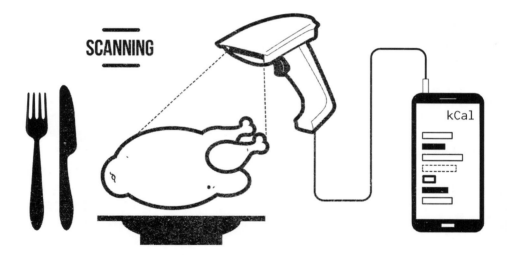

SCANNING

kCal

WHAT WOULD HAPPEN IF PATIENTS LED HEALTHCARE?

#hcsm #epatient #hcldr #patientvoice | Extraordinary Measures (2010)

I have been asked this question twice. The wording was the same both times but the circumstances and the tone were very different. I gave a workshop in Paris about what to do with the digital world as a medical professional. I brought up the topic of empowering patients and how doing so will change the way we practice medicine. At the end a physician asked the question above in a very sarcastic tone.

The second time happened in Austria at the Salzburg Global Seminars that challenge leaders to tackle issues of global concern. A public health researcher asked me this question and seemed very interested in the answer. As it turned out she wanted to bring the concept of patient empowerment to her home country in Africa.

I have never talked about patients leading healthcare. I have spoken about patients leading their own care. These are different things, but I still had to provide reasonable and persuasive answers to them. The irritated physician thought that letting patients lead healthcare or even their own care was unworkable. After all there is a reason why training physicians takes more than a decade at the minimum. The African researcher by contrast thought it would be a new perspective in their healthcare system. Currently all decisions are driven by physicians, but she saw the point in letting patients control what happens to them.

This is where two schools of thought collide. One assumes the superiority and authority of physicians over all medical decisions. The other sees the wisdom in empowering patients. The latter is a relatively new perspective given that the ability to access health records and resources only become available in the past decade or so, as have small devices that measure health parameters in private. Dr. Tom Ferguson founder of e–patients.net, said that „e–Patients are Empowered, Engaged, Equipped and Enabled." That is where the "e" comes from, but I believe we will stop using the expression because soon every patient will be empowered. Why would not they be? They can access resources and medical devices. Why wouldn't they actively participate in their care?

Some of them don't want to. Most are not encouraged by their caregivers to participate in a therapeutic partnership. A prominent proponent of empowerment is e–Patient Dave deBronkart from the US. He told me his life was saved by the best scientific medicine at an academic medical center coupled with practical advice from fellow patients with no training in the biology of his disease. It took centuries for medicine to reach today's standards, and the science has produced results that sometimes look miraculous. But not only biological knowledge is useful.

DeBronkart thinks that scientific experts, the clinical experts, and patients and their families should be at the same table. As if to confirm his point of view, deBronkart was invited as a Visiting Professor in 2015 by Internal Medicine Chief Residents at the Mayo Clinic.

The real future shift will be about health, prevention, and early detection. Physicians and policy makers may think the ordinary adult is not responsible enough to guide their own health, but just think how motivated parents can be about their young children, and how motivated adults are to look after their elders' well–being. Offering those caregivers convenient and time–saving technology will gain adoption quickly.

When I asked deBronkart to answer the initial question he said that if patients led healthcare then prevention would be at the top of the list. It would be easy to do as would monitoring for early detection.

His physician, Dr. Danny Sands, says that healthcare by definition involves a professional who is paid for care delivered and is legally responsible for management and outcome. When practiced properly healthcare should be a collaboration between patient and caregiver. There is an enormous place for self–care, but when the professional becomes involved it is best done as a collaborator and only rarely as an unquestioned authority. Physician leaders in the 21st century care very much about patient autonomy.

Both patient and physician bring important things to the table. The physician brings years of knowledge and experience, and hopefully some wisdom. Patients contribute as experts in themselves. Because it is a collaboration neither party is "in charge". Patients should not demand things from their providers, but engage in reasoned conversation. This is why Dr. Sands doesn't prescribe tests or medications to people just because they ask for them. He advocates that every medical practice and hospital have a role for patients and families such as the engaged Patient and Family Advisory Council at his practice.

In 2014 the prestigious British Medical Journal promoted patient partnerships as important to improving quality, safety, cost effectiveness, and sustainability of healthcare in Great Britain. They encouraged authors of educational articles to co–produce their papers with patients or have them describe the nature of their involvement. It also meant including patient reviews of submitted papers in their customary peer review processes, and appointing patients and patient advocates to the journal's editorial board. In recognition the British Medical Journal was the first publication to receive a "Patients Included" certificate.

The award has gone to events and organizations that invite patients as speakers or members of the advisory board. Academic medicine needs their insights, but how can patients help if they don't own their own medical data?

Hugo Campos, a visual designer and creative director, became famous for his fight to obtain the data generated by his implanted defibrillator. His life depends on the device. After he lost his health insurance the defibrillator's manufacturer denied him the data. As a Quantified Self man who wants to measure parameters of his health, Campos paid to take a course on cardiac rhythm management and purchased a pacemaker programmer on eBay. This gave him access to the implant and restored his autonomy and right to self–protection, as he himself claimed. Actually he might be the only pacemaker–defibrillator patient with the ability to interrogate his own implant.

He thinks patients will never lead healthcare, or rather "disease care" as he puts it, but patients will continue to expand their role in self–care where they can exercise their autonomy. Patients will continue to ask for technology solutions that enhance their autonomy, and the physician's role will shift to solving complex problems and performing difficult interventions.

The new vision of healthcare is participatory. What would happen if patients led healthcare? It would not work just like how it doesn't work if physicians are leading healthcare alone. Patients should be at the center of care and attention. They should be experts of their own health, and medical professionals should be experts of their fields. Patients should own and get access to their own data. One promising example is the Blue Button movement in the US that lets patients download their medical records. With or without technology, physicians should encourage their patients toward more self–care either, and learn how to transform frustrated patients into e–patients. Does it sound Utopian? No. It has already been happening.

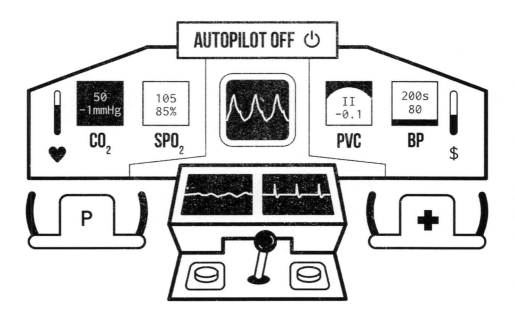

CAN I IMPROVE MY BRAIN?

#QS #brainweek #brainhealth | Limitless (2011) Lucy (2014)

Every semester I am invited by the Department of Behavioral Sciences at Semmelweis Medical School in Budapest to speak to first–year medical students. They have just started the semester and here I come telling them how technology will transform their work and why they won't have a job unless they acquire skills relevant to the digital world. I wish someone had told me this when I was a beginning medical student.

I show my wearable devices to give them an idea of what to expect when they start practicing medicine. I also talk about empowering patients and how the responsibility of caregivers will change from what it is now. The students seem to enjoy hearing this, and after seeing the variety of wearables that patients can access I thought they would want to explore the ethical issues. Instead, one student wanted to know whether it was possible to improve his brain.

I assumed he meant improving mental skills without resorting to pills. Skills such as mental flexibility, problem solving, attention, and memory. Students have to incorporate a huge amount of information during their education. This ranges from hard facts to the art of practicing medicine. Then they continue to learn throughout their career which can span five decades. Anything that can aid this lifetime learning is an asset. Technology can help with that.

The Muse headband has seven sensors, five on the forehead and one behind each ear, that measure brain activity which users can see charted on a smartphone. It translates the measured EEG into a graph anyone without experience with EEG can understand. During relaxation sessions, users listen to beach sounds that change depending on how relaxed they are. Getting such immediate feedback helps individuals how to relax themselves. The Interaxon company behind Muse is working with tens of thousands of users and universities worldwide to find ways to assist students in studying. If students see how their attention changes during studying sessions, they might be able to choose the best times to study more efficiently.

Lumosity is a service providing web–based and mobile games with neuroscientists in their team. Games are claimed to improve mental flexibility, focus, or short–term memory. Lumosity had 50 million members in 2014. Users have played games over a billion times, and more than 280,000 people participated in studies launched by the company. In my experience, it improved my attention and memory. It is also a great way to start my day. I must note the caveat, however, that any activity such as Lumosity, playing cards, meditating, or walking in the woods in which you practice staying on task will help your attention span and focus, and thus other cognitive tasks that depend on them.

Melon developed a different headband that combines measurements and games. The band gives instant feedback about the user's state of focus by using brainwave monitoring. It sends data wirelessly to a smartphone and teaches the user how to get better by playing games. In sessions that take about 6 minutes, the color of the background represents the level of attention while one is playing these games.

Thync received the Top Tech of CES 2015 Award in the Cool Tech category. It uses signaling in the form of electrical pulses delivered through programs they call Vibes. There are two types of vibes. Calm Vibes help the brain relax; Energy Vibes give an energy boost. The user selects what kind of Vibes they should receive to reach an energized, relaxed, or focused state of mind. This employs energy levels within the normal range of brain activity using advanced bio–materials. The company claims to work within FDA guidelines to maintain regulatory compliance although it has not been approved yet. They also claim that peer–reviewed studies support the idea behind their technology, but as of 2015, there is no study mentioning the device or its effectiveness.

Halo Neuroscience looked into this idea further. They have attempted to create a headband that improves cognitive skills by shocking the brain with electric currents. The science behind this is far from proven. Nonetheless is backed by a $1,5 million investment from Marc Andreessen, inventor of the modern web browser. Halo invited test users to its San Francisco office in May, 2015. Malcolm Gladwell, as he said in *Outliers: The Story of Success,* estimates that 10,000 hours of practice are required to achieve mastery of any demanding skill such as playing the violin. The team behind Halo claims that number can be reduced. If practicing a skill becomes more efficient because of immediate feedback, that feedback might hasten the process of mastery. They believe that with their device people could become an expert athlete or musician in fewer than 10,000 hours. Of course they have not tested this supposition, but time will tell. We sorely need persuasive evidence coming from methodologically well–designed studies that either support or refute their speculations.

Open–Source Brain–Computer Interface (OpenBCI) is an ad–hoc cohort of researchers, engineers, artists, and designers who hope to channel the electrical signals of the body and brain. Their sensor samples electrical brain activity (EEG), muscle activity (EMG), and heart activity (ECG).

CEO Conor Russomanno told me that my medical student was prescient in his question because personalized neurofeedback training is a real and growing enterprise. A number of commercial EEG–based applications such as Muse, Emotiv, Neurosky, and OpenBCI purport to aid people in mindfulness training and their ability to meditate and focus. This contrasts with services such as Lumosity and Quantified Mind that don't require a physical device and are geared towards improving memory or attention.

He believes we have still not reached the peak of what is possible with emerging technologies for recording biometric data in a real world context. We have had a big push with respect to hardware devices. Now software has to catch up so we can get full value from them. An interesting possibility will be the merging of EEG–based devices with augmented reality, virtual reality, and wearables.

Technology can play a role in relaxing and improving our brain. What if cognitive performance became a factor in landing a job? People might resort to smart drugs and the memory enhancers already available and known as nootropic drugs. Surveys find that 3% to 11% of American students and about 5% of German ones have taken cognitive enhancers in their lifetime. These percentages are growing.

After smart drugs and wearable devices, more advanced technologies will follow. For instance, the US Defense Advanced Research Projects Agency (DARPA) and also IBM built a microchip whose architecture is inspired by the neuronal structure of the brain in that it requires only a minuscule fraction of the electrical power consumed by conventional chips. These chips can be tied together like tiles and simulate neural networks. There might come an era of brain implants that improve long–term cognitive function. The problem is that it's hard to implant anything in the brain without damaging it, and the implant material must be biocompatible.

The one atom thick graphene can serve as a solution. In 2014, graphene implants allowed researchers to instigate limb movements in mice by using light. This method, called optogenetics, makes it possible to activate or deactivate a small group of brain cells with unprecedented precision. Human applications are light–years away though.

It may become increasingly more difficult to keep our brains technology–free. Keeping a healthy balance between leaving our mind as it is and improving it with technology is challenging. But I imagine that anyone who tries such a device may discover that the options are well worth the effort.

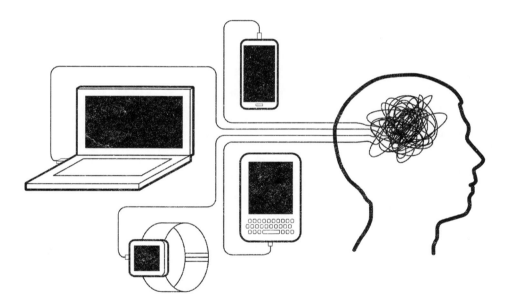

CAN SOCIAL MEDIA HELP PREVENT AND NOTIFY ABOUT EPIDEMICS?

#hcsm #globalhealth #publichealth | 12 Monkeys (1995) Contagion (2011)

Out of a global population of 7.2 billion as of 2015, about 3 billion people have access to the Internet. Of these 2 billion have social media accounts such as Facebook or Twitter. Around 3.6 billion people own mobile phones and 1.6 billion of those access social media from it. These numbers are increasing even as we talk about them. Social media channels could become the perfect infrastructure for gathering and disseminating information. Each day, there are 4.5 billion likes on Facebook. 500 million Twitter messages are sent. 70 million photos and videos are uploaded to Instagram. The list goes on.

Social media is the information highway in my life, too. Through my professional networks on Linkedin, Facebook, and Twitter I maintain contact with experts in my field. Social media lets me not feel isolated. I have built a whole system for how to get the information I need and how to spread the word when it's needed. Organizers of a TEDx event in the Netherlands invited me to talk about that. I described how the experts on my Linkedin or Facebook channels filter the news for me, and how I once crowdsourced a complicated diagnosis by using Twitter.

No questions are permitted after a TEDx talk, but during the reception afterwards a professor of public health approached me. She didn't use many digital tools in her work, but wanted to know more about how I got the most out of my social networks. She then asked if social media could help prevent and warn about epidemics. Knowing how big the 2014 Ebola outbreak in Western Africa was, this is a timely question.

On September 30, 2014 the first reports came out about a Liberian man at a Dallas hospital being diagnosed with Ebola. By October 1, 6000 Twitter messages a minute were being sent about Ebola. Studies show that people are more likely to trust information that comes from people they know than from faceless organizations. And so a single false statement on Twitter can affect thousands because it is so widely taken as fact. This is why public health organizations have been conscientiously building their online presence. They want to reach people more effectively.

The US Centers for Disease Control and Prevention (CDC) operates a social media platform in multiple languages that covers an enormous range of topics from flu and smoking cessation to emergencies and chronic diseases. The World Health Organization (WHO) also has similar social media accounts.

The first well–known effort to predict an outbreak was attempted by Google in 2008. By aggregating Google search queries that mentioned flu symptoms, it attempted to predict flu outbreaks in the US. Later, it extended the effort to twenty–five countries. The earlier the warning about an outbreak is available, the earlier that prevention measures can be enacted. At first the Google Flu Trends overestimated outbreaks. Studies concluded that it wasn't as accurate as the CDC's surveillance programs. But with ever–improving algorithms it has the potential to assist organizations in making very accurate predictions.

People don't just search for symptoms of an infectious disease on Google. They unwittingly help spread an alert by retweeting and sharing posts on Facebook. In an ideal world relevant data would pour constantly into a server of a public health organization. Smart algorithms would then analyze it and alert us about an epidemic before it even happened. We can think of social media as sensors of a big data system. Such a system would be better than randomly monitoring actual sick people, as many offline studies do.

Twitter is also a good channel for reaching out. Researchers like it because it is fast. New infections might not even appear in CDC statistics until the patient goes to the hospital or does something else that causes the ailment to be reported. Twitter is not that accurate, but is fast. People can report cases the moment they wake up with a sore throat. Twitter also provides geographical locations.

We need to get the most out of this hive of information. Algorithms must distinguish between a new case of flu and people merely talking about flu when a football player, say, misses a match because of a fever. Becoming better at understanding context could yield really good predictions. Eventually, these new methods will exceed those that are currently used.

Epidemics are not just about infectious diseases. They cover all kinds of conditions that are socially contagious such as dieting, or psychological disorders as anxiety. Properly designed social media channels could mine such information. Privacy concerns should be a priority, and information must be anonymous. Social media channels are perhaps going in this direction.

When the devastating Nepal earthquake happened in April, 2015 Facebook was able to test a feature they had rolled out months before. Safety Check let people tell their friends and family that they are fine. 7 million people used it in the wake of the earthquake, almost a quarter of Nepal's population.

By encouraging users to make donations, Facebook also raised more than $10 million for relief efforts.

Being connected to each other is amazing. If the safety and privacy issues are taken care of with enough efforts, social media can revolutionize public health. Until then, keep on tweeting.

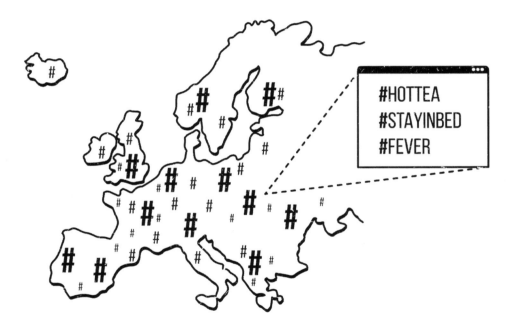

COULD WE TRAIN DOCTORS THE WAY DUOLINGO TEACHES LANGUAGE?

#meded #hcsmcourse #MOOCs | The Doctor (1991)

Medical education doesn't prepare students for the world they will face when they start practicing medicine. The amount of medical information is growing at an almost exponential pace. Patients now communicate through social media. Disruptive technology has reached healthcare. The status quo must change. To address this I launched a course about social media, mobile health, and innovations at Semmelweis Medical School some years ago. I made the curriculum available online and threw in a pinch of gaming. Over 10,000 physicians have since completed the online course. That's not enough. Every future physician worldwide should be adept in the digital world.

Before I served on a PhD dissertation committee in the Netherlands in 2014, I spent 2 hours talking about this with Jur Koksma, an assistant professor and education expert. When we came to a point of having to come up with an example of how to teach a skill we both valued highly, we each said "Duolingo" at the same time.

I have been using the Duolingo smartphone application for over a year. I wanted to learn Spanish, but have no time to visit a teacher or take classes. But I was willing to dedicate a few minutes to learning Spanish every day. That's how I bumped into Duolingo. You download it for free, select what language you want to learn, and jump in immediately. Duolingo doesn't go into grammatical rules and exceptions. It just asks you to play. Eventually you will learn the language. Duolingo has over 60 million users and covers more than 20 languages.

It teaches a language by providing extensive written lessons, and practice in dictation and speaking. The part I like best is a gamified skill tree through which users can progress. A vocabulary section helps you memorize words, and a crowdsourced platform familiarizes you with translation. The latter is at the heart of Duolingo's business model. The app is free, but it crowdsources translations for companies such as CNN and Buzzfeed.

Users gain experience points and learn skills as they use the app. It remembers what mistakes the user made and brings the material up often for practice. It takes about 34 hours on Duolingo to yield the same reading and writing ability as a freshman college semester that takes more than 130 hours.

I like Duolingo not because of what it teaches but because of how it teaches. Combining gaming, rewards, and community is brilliant. It may be possible to drive medical learning by using Duolingo–like apps. Studies have shown that self–testing is far more efficient than just reading textbooks. Combined with group learning among medical students the approach promises many benefits.

At the University of Helsinki and the George Washington University, each freshman medical student is given an iPad loaded with digital reference books and course materials. In the program that launched in 2011, students also receive a digital package containing textbooks, apps and study materials, all in digital format. At these universities, and others, the curriculum has become virtually paperless. At George Washington University small learning groups of ten students also work with a reference librarian during the semester who teaches them how to navigate databases and find the information they need. We are training a new generation of Internet–savvy doctors.

These approaches could eliminate the need for traditional exams given that one can continually evaluate a student's progress and accumulation of knowledge. The skills imparted are more related to real life contexts than those learned in old format in which they had to perform on subjective exams at specific times during the semester.

Massive open online courses, or MOOCs, are scalable in size and accessible to far flung audiences. Khan Academy, Coursera, Edx, and Udacity instruct students around the world about basic topics as well as highly advanced issues. Anyone has access to world–class lectures at Stanford or Yale on YouTube. The ability to access the very best knowledge and wisdom has never been greater.

The Australian Monash University prints out anatomical structures in 3D when there are cadaver shortages. Anatomage developed a digital dissection table on which students can dissect the human body from multiple angles. Live videos of operations can be accessed on ORlive.com. The New York University School of Medicine designed a virtual microscope to let students learn histology and pathology. Interactive virtual bodies, medical quizzes, apps describing case presentations, and many more educational tools are accessible to students worldwide. Such digital solutions should support, but not substitute current medical curriculum. When the current generation of physicians starts teaching the next one, they will need real experience.

The primary goal of the medical curriculum is to train great medical professionals. Practicing medicine today entails using more and more technology, and so physicians need to become expert in using these tools too. Preparation should begin in medical school. If we do not change how physicians are trained for the future, medical students will individually adjust to the new needs finding their own ways. This is not the solution we need.

Today's medical curriculum is designed in a way that it can only slowly change. Its methods are outdated. Better ones that use gaming are already available. It is time to let students enjoy studying medicine and the process of becoming a doctor.

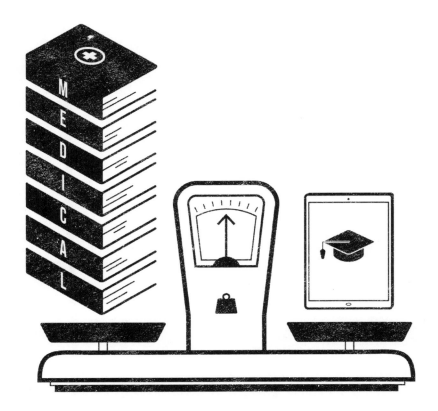

WILL ROBOTS TAKE OVER OUR JOBS IN HEALTHCARE?

#robotics #robots | I, Robot (2004) Moon (2009) Humans (2015)

I teach another course about the future of healthcare to medical, public health, and allied students. In one lecture I ask students to design the future of care. They come up with their own ideas. We talk them through those and design the process of care in real time. Doing this I learn a lot each semester about how students think about the future. I had an older student with a previous degree in economics. He had decided to become a doctor at the age of 30. When I spoke about what jobs robots and algorithms might take in the future, he raised his hand and asked whether robots would take over our jobs in healthcare—with a very worried look on his face.

Surgical robots become increasingly precise each day. Man–size robots can lift and move patients and transport them throughout the hospital. I held a PARO therapeutic robot in my arms. It was cute and calmed me. At a conference I once watched how a diminutive robot made an entire audience dance with it. It only takes the Xenex robot 10 minutes to disinfect a patient room with UV light. A robot called Tug works at hospitals in the San Francisco Bay Area. It delivers food and medicine. It picks up waste and laundry. It navigates the halls without crashing into people.

Robots are more common in other industries than in healthcare. The BakeBot robot serves customers fresh cookies. A robot named Baxter can beat any human at the popular game Connect Four. Another robot can continuously rearrange solar panels so that they always follow the sun. Robots are becoming more human–like and more affordable, although we must wait for a robot companion we can have at home that lives up to expectations.

That student asked about robots, but I think he was really asking about automation. Automation includes robotic devices, robots that look like a human, and algorithms. Silicon Valley investor Vinod Khosla once said something that resonated within the medical community for a long time. He said that technology would replace 80% of doctors because machines, driven by big data and computational power, would not only be cheaper but more accurate and objective than the average doctor. He added that we eventually wouldn't need doctors at all.

In 2015 the information technology research firm Gartner predicted that one–third of existing jobs will be replaced by software, robots, and smart machines by 2025. Blue collar as well as white collar workers such as financial and sports reporters, marketers, surgeons, and financial analysts were in danger of being replaced. As Martin Ford outlines in *Rise of the Robots*, healthcare represented less than 6% in the US economy in 1960. Its share had tripled by 2013. The real issue is not utilizing too many robots but too few. Typically robots are expensive but reduce costs. Medicine and healthcare won't be able to and should not try to avoid this.

Google has acquired a number of robotics companies. Apple has so far spent $10.5 billion on them. Amazon acquired Kiva Systems for $750 million in order to further automate its warehouses. In 2014, 200,000 industrial robots were installed, 15% more than in 2013. The use of robotics in the electronics industry is cheaper than new hires, costing $4 per hour compared to an average hourly wage of $9–10.

If we look at the history of automation the first wave of machines in the 19th century was better at assembling things than people were. The second wave machines were better at organizing things. Today data analytics, cognitive computers, and self–driving cars suggest that they are better at pattern–recognition.

But both the simplest tasks and the most complicated ones require people. By simplest I mean that there is a greater chance a robot can play chess than go upstairs. By complicated I mean that regarding jobs such as managers, healthcare workers, and others related to education or media; humans are still superior at working with, and caring for others humans. Although, making a diagnosis is cheaper with cognitive computers than doing that alone as physicians.

But whether a robot can make an ethical decision is a huge question. An interesting experiment raised this issue. In it a small robot was programmed not to let other robots called human proxies, which represented real people, get into the danger zone on a table game. When only one human proxy approached the danger zone, the robot could successfully thwart it. But when two proxies appeared the robot became confused, and in 14 out of 33 trials it wasted so much time trying to decide that both human proxies fell into the hole. Robots cannot make yet the ethical decisions that characterize experienced physicians.

Automation will make the world better and create opportunities for people clever enough to seize them. But healthcare will change. Tasks and procedures that can be automated should be, and will be. Algorithms will make diagnoses based on quantifiable data better than how humans do it now alone. It is easy to automate the fabrication of equipment or the transportation of patients. The challenge comes when empathy and interpersonal interaction comes into play. Robots won't approach this level of sophistication for a long time.

To answer my initial question: many jobs will be taken over by robots and automation in the coming years. If people whose jobs are replaced cannot acquire new skills or improve their existing ones, they will no longer have a job. Given this possibility we must constantly question what our best individual skills are and what we can do to improve them. Let's make sure to attend to those skills that make us irreplaceable.

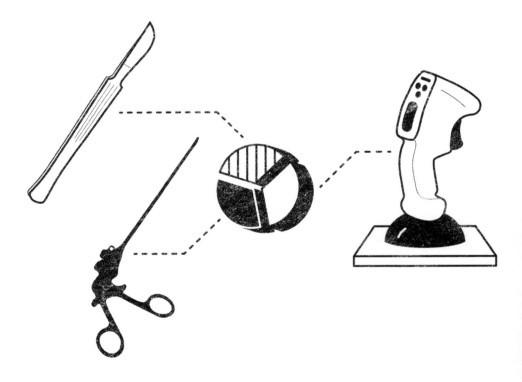

WHEN WILL WE FIND THE CURE FOR CANCER?

#cancer #BCSM #LCSM | 50/50 (2011) The Fault In Our Stars (2014) Self/less (2015)

I spoke at a conference in the Netherlands at which patients were not only included in the program but also in the organizing committee. After my talk a patient said that there were many incidents of cancer in her family. She wanted to know when we would find a cure. Her tone suggested that she was optimistic one would be found eventually. But she was not happy with my answer.

I told her that every patient's cancer is unique. Each of us is genetically different from others and thus reacts to diseases in an idiosyncratic way. I told her that every cancer was also genetically different. Finding a "cure for cancer" implies that cancer is a single disease. But it is not.

Cell types from blood to skin regularly grow and duplicate. The process is controlled by a complicated molecular switch. Normally, if a cell begins to multiply uncontrollably, defense mechanisms make it kill itself, or the immune system removes it before it turns into cancerous tissue. Plenty of types of cells become uncontrollable every day, but a healthy immune system can deal with it. The problem occurs when either cells outgrow everything else at a rapid pace, or when the immune system cannot cope with it. Genetic predispositions and environmental factors also play a part, but in only a few cancer types can we identify a single cause.

Modern medicine has strived to describe the background of cancer for decades. After cardiovascular diseases it is the leading cause of death worldwide. Lung scans, tumor markers in the blood, and simple dermatological tests can all identify cancer at an early stage. But not all cancer types cause symptoms or can be detected early.

Early cancer detection can be based either on molecular features or symptoms. Imagine if specific blood tests became so inexpensive that it would be worth checking them on a regular basis. Or perhaps nanorobots swimming in our bloodstream could keep an eye on this constantly.

Another approach is developing treatments that can either assist the immune system or target cancerous cells directly. The former is promising, but greater effort has been put into the latter. Therapies have been designed that target cancerous tissue based on its genetic composition. In breast cancer, for example, the cells of certain patients express a protein called HER–2 on the surface. A drug has been developed to attack those cells. For patients who do not express this protein, the drug is ineffective.

Tissue from a lung cancer patient can be genetically analyzed today, and treatment options selected on the basis of its genetic background. This is personalized medicine at its most refined. Because cancer cells replicate much faster than other cells, they survive through natural selection played out on a small scale. Tumors become resistant to drugs that used to be efficient. When this happens a new genetic analysis is necessary to find a new treatment that the cancer is sensitive to. This kind of targeted therapy is very expensive and not available to the broad population.

What makes it expensive is the drawn out process pharmaceutical companies need to go through in order to get an FDA approved drug. It costs billions of dollars and takes more than a decade to accomplish. But if clinical trials became more digital and genetic analysis more affordable, then costs would fall.

Chemotherapy is a broad shotgun: it attacks all cells including normal as well as cancerous ones that grow and duplicate. This is why chemotherapy has such nasty side effects such as hair loss, a weakened immune system, and susceptibility to otherwise innocuous infections. A longstanding goal has been to make chemotherapy target only cells that are cancerous. So far this has proven impossible, and the targeted genetic approach above is prohibitively expensive. Another approach is to fashion drug molecules so that they reach only cancer cells and do not interfere with normal ones. To attempt this, nanotechnology has fashioned tiny cages that enclose active drug molecules. The premise is that such cages could enter the cancerous cells and thus spare normal ones from the drug's toxic effects.

We have about 24,000 genes, only 500 of which have any relation to cancer. But within those 500 genes one can find about 2 million unique errors related to cancer and billions of possible combinations that such gene errors can have with one another. This is what makes developing cancer drugs maddeningly tricky. These numbers might seem shocking, but a new generation of devices that can make the code of the DNA quickly available has brought a revolution to oncology. There are approximately forty to fifty targeted drugs now available, and current clinical trials investigate about 200 potential targets. This means that the hope for finding targeted therapies is increasing every day.

Cancer is not just about finding effective treatments. Dealing with cancer is sometimes a decades–long affair. Patients need ongoing emotional and social support, and here is where the long–tail effect of social media comes in. Patients who have a rare disease are unlikely to meet like–minded individuals where they live. But finding them online is quite possible.

Online community sites such as Inspire or Smart Patients have been around for years. In these communities patients share medical issues with one another as well as personal stories. As e–Patient Dave deBronkart said, besides the medical advice his doctor gave him, interaction with fellow patients was an enormous help.

The real goal is to make cancer a short bump in life instead of a life event that might lead to death. We won't cure cancer as one disease, but we have better technologies to make the life event to bump transformation happen. Until then, keep an eye on the alarming symptoms.

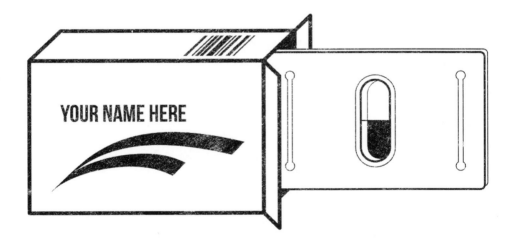

WILL DOCTORS ALWAYS HAVE TO SEE PATIENTS IN PERSON?

#digitalhealth #telemedicine / Logan's Run (1976)

A telecommunications company in the Netherlands invited me to give an after dinner talk to executives. There is charm in speaking after 9 p.m. when people are well fed and relaxed. I talked about how smartphones, tablets, and telemedicine devices were about to disrupt healthcare. I mentioned Uber, and how its model could be partially applied to healthcare. The executives were intrigued. Will physicians always have to see patients in person? The question was not whether doctors will continue to see patients in person, but whether they will have to.

The essence of care is the face–to–face meeting of physician and patient. Increasingly, this is becoming a luxury. We cannot train enough doctors to meet growing global demand. Additionally, as medicine has become more complicated, training has become more intense and takes more time. The increasing gap may never be filled in the traditional way. For example, Africa has 28% of the world's disease burden but only 3% of the healthcare workforce. Telemedicine can both supplement and substitute for traditional doctor–patient interactions.

The aim of technology is not to remove in–person visits when they otherwise could take place, but to make it possible for the patient to access a doctor. Even when telemedicine is used in a clinic an attending nurse or doctor is usually present along with the remote specialist.

The directors of InTouch Health, a company developing remote care solutions and devices, told me about a family living in a remote area of Bolivia. A child had been ill for eighteen years without ever having received a concrete diagnosis. After a remote consultation with a medical team in Saskatchewan that lasted only 45 minutes, the adolescent's problem was properly identified. The family can sleep soundly now knowing that there is hope and a treatment that will change their lives for the better.

In another case a 60 year–old Cleveland woman collapsed while doing laundry in her basement. She crawled up the stairs and phoned for help. An ambulance arrived 20 minutes later and did a CT scan. A neurologist at the Cleveland Clinic remotely read the results, diagnosed a stroke, and the mobile team started appropriate treatment 32 minutes after the patient entered the van. With stroke, treatment as soon as possible is crucial to prevent permanent injury. Remote access to a specialist turned out to be decisive in this case.

And yet there are many things physicians cannot yet do remotely. We cannot smell, even though that can sometimes be diagnostic. We cannot touch, although sensors that would let us feel what another person feels at a distance are in the making. Smartphone cameras are not always well balanced and the lighting conditions are not ideal. Yet there is no reason not to expect that improvements are underway.

Services turned to the model of Uber to create a business model for on-demand visits in person. The company called Firstline offers doctor visits through a smartphone application. The patient can choose among the specialists and whether they need a call, a text message or the house call. Similarly to Uber, if there is a doctor in the neighborhood, the visit can take place soon and prescriptions are sent electronically to the local pharmacy. Teleconsultation has a monthly fee and house calls have a one-time fee that can be reimbursed by some insurance companies.

A Chicago-based startup, Go2Nurse, applies the physician model for remote access to nurses. There are hundreds of registered nurses in the metropolitan area. Patients can request home service and pay through the app just like in Uber. Patients have the option of chatting with a nurse first to find out whether the house call is warranted. The app can also translate from English to Spanish.

Other examples are available worldwide. In Indonesia Philips is running a pilot project that helps doctors remotely monitor pregnant women. Data obtained remotely are sent via mobile phone to obstetricians who can determine whether a pregnancy is high risk of not. In Kenya, 12,000 nurses learned how to treat major diseases such as HIV and malaria through an e-learning project. It trained more nurses than any physical classroom could handle. The Jordan Healthcare Initiative uses Cisco HealthPresence technology to expand the reach of specialty healthcare to rural communities in Jordan.

Hawaii was one of the first places where residents could pay a flat fee for a ten-minute doctor visit online or by phone. Video consultation will become part of routine healthcare, removing unnecessary patient visits from the system. Think of the number of days missed from work for no reason except traveling and waiting times. Think of the anxiety people go through waiting to get medical attention. Most of us live with smartphones, which are the gateway towards this solution. The technology is already there. We need now good business models and services.

Patients with skin lesions can snap a photo with their phone, fill out a short questionnaire, and submit it to a Swedish service, iDoc24. They receive an answer within 24 hours for a one–time fee. CellScope developed a smartphone that can take a quality picture of the ear canal. When a patient suspects ear infection, they submit the picture to the service and get remote medical help. Most companies that provide such services claim they do not provide medical advice but rather educational information. This is a way to skirt regulations, and is not likely to change until government regulations do.

Remote care exists not only between caregivers and households, but also within clinical settings. InTouch Health's robots can safely navigate around the clinic and provide remote video consultation. At some clinics such robots have become routine members of the staff. In US supermarkets specially designed booths allow patients to submit their vital signs and talk to a physician via video.

These developments will lead to the increasing use of virtual reality devices. Patients will be able to experience 3D interaction with a remote doctor. Only human touch will be missing from the visit, but textiles and gloves with tactile feedback might eventually make it possible to feel what the other person feels from the distant location.

Telemedicine promises to bridge the space between delivery of care and people who have no access to it. Technologies with viable business models could deliver care where it has not been available before. Paradoxical as it may sound; digital approaches could actually spread the human touch.

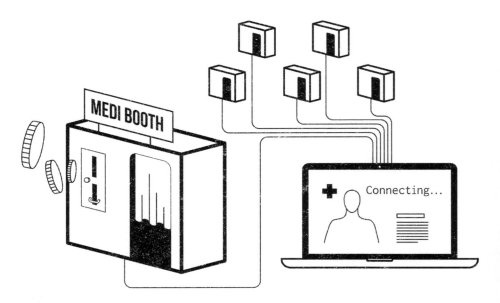

WILL INNOVATIVE MEDICAL TECHNOLOGY BE ACCESSIBLE TO THE POOR?

#digitalhealth | Elysium (2013)

This question has come up at two different events: at a public health round-table in Barcelona, and at a digital health conference in Dubai. Financial inequalities are always a struggle, but growing inequalities in health may well cause chaos. If we remain optimistic, disruptive technologies will decrease the cost of care delivery. But this will only happen if there is a strong societal demand to improve those devices and services.

Organizations and forward–thinking individuals have come up with ideas for how to improve the conditions of those living in underdeveloped areas. Mick Ebeling, CEO of Not Impossible, met a boy named Daniel in Sudan who had had both his arms blown off. Ebeling decided to print out a customized prosthetic hand–the start of the famous Project Daniel. Ebeling also trained local people how to print out prostheses for other amputees. He hopes that Daniel's story will initiate a global effort.

E–Nable similarly makes prosthetic hands for kids by using 3D printers. It costs around $25 to print out the parts. A restored hand allows kids to ride a bicycle, pick up a glass, or play with other kids. With a $600,000 grant from Google and a partnership with 3DSystems, E–Nable was able to distribute inexpensive prosthetics to those in need worldwide. I examined their adult prosthetic hand in Paris at the Doctors 2.0 and You event and I was surprised with its grip and overall structure even though it had been manufactured in hours from printed 3D elements.

Another example is SonoSite that developed a mobile ultrasound technology providing diagnostic–quality imaging to any locations. An organization called Floating Doctors set up a mobile clinic in the village community of Bahia Grande on the Panama coastline. The first physician to use this technology performed a gallbladder scan on an elderly woman with abdominal pain at her home.

Coupling such innovations with people who are willing to help in underdeveloped areas might counterintuitively provide faster access to care than patients living in developed countries. Lack of local regulations and urgent need for services bring this about.

With the hospital coming to our homes via wearable gadgets and telemedicine, it will gradually become less relevant whether a patient lives within a developed or underdeveloped healthcare system. The rapid penetration of mobile phone service puts the device that is needed to establish a digital connection already in patients' hands.

The Global Impact Competitions organized by the Singularity University serve this goal. The competitions serve to identify outstanding entrepreneurs, leaders, scientists, and engineers who have the most forward–looking ideas that can affect millions of lives within the next 3 to 5 years. Winners of the local events receive a full scholarship for their Graduate Program. Past winning applications include an image processing technology to categorize and monitor chronic wounds; an autonomous RoboSweeper vehicle for collecting and processing garbage; and a gaming platform called Harimata for detecting and tracking autism and learning disabilities.

The Visioneering division of XPrize aims to identify future problems concerning food, health, and home that can be solved through prize competitions. The Bill & Melinda Gates Foundation oversees a Global Heath Program that works to improve health conditions in developing countries. Current projects address malaria, HIV, pneumonia, and tuberculosis.

The cost of medical technology has been rising for decades, and it is the driving force behind the developments I've been discussing. Disruptive innovations can reverse the upward cost trend. In 2003 a 128 MB USB drive cost about $35, the price of a 128 GB drive in 2015. Solar cells in 1977 cost $70 per Watt. By 2013 it had dropped to $0.74 per Watt. Laparoscopic surgery frees up hospital operating rooms. By definition a disruptive technology always gets cheaper compared to traditional ones.

Another driving force bringing costs down is crowdfunding. Silicon Valley entrepreneurs came up with an idea for a small device that laypeople can use to measure their vital signs. Scanadu launched a crowdfunding campaign in 2013, and received $1.66 million from 8,800 backers on Indiegogo.com. After it shipped the first devices they started getting more attention and more funding. As of May, 2015 they have around $50 million in capitalization.

We can decrease healthcare costs by letting Moore's law, the exponential improvement of technology, take care of it. We cannot make traditional healthcare less expensive without lessening the burden on it by having people develop healthier habits now. That is honestly not going to happen. What does need to happen is establishing a new climate for companies willing and able to disrupt healthcare costs. Research finds that only 0.5% of studies evaluated new technologies that work just as well as existing ones but cost less. The more society demands that this change, the sooner it will happen.

Jaundice affects about 9 million newborns in developing countries. The cure is simple: blue light. But the phototherapy lamps cost upward of $3,000. A non–profit design firm called D–Rev made such a device for only $350. In the tests conducted by Stanford University, the new machines out-performed the traditional and more expensive ones.

In developing countries wheelchairs must deal with rough roads. But equipment that can handle rough terrain is expensive, between $2,000 and $5,000 per chair. MIT's Mobility Lab designed a leveraged chair that could handle off–road conditions for $200.

Sanitary pads are not always accessible to women living in underde-veloped areas, and they are expensive. They might skip about 50 work and school days every year because they need to stay at home while menstruat-ing. An MIT graduate developed a machine that can make pads from banana pulp. Disruptive ideas now come fast to areas where there is great need.

In Ghana, Nigeria, Kenya, and Tanzania, patients can text the code on the label of a malaria drug to a free number and receive an immediate yes or no whether the drug is genuine or counterfeit.

With an Internet connection the range of opportunities for anyone who wants to change a system is wider than ever. Crowdsourcing informa-tion from experts around the globe, crowdfunding for a good idea, or using a local 3D printer to manufacture a prototype all make it possible for people in underdeveloped areas to sometimes design better medical tools than those in Silicon Valley or Europe can.

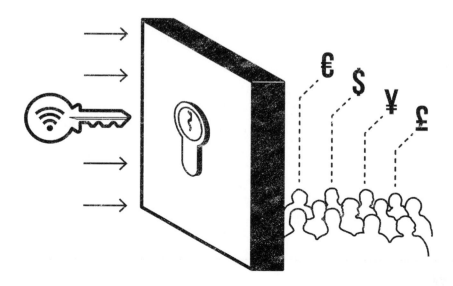

HOW WILL TECHNOLOGY TRANSFORM THE FUTURE OF SPORT?

#digitalhealth #sport | Back To The Future (1985) Real Steel (2011)

The Dean of the University of Physical Education in Budapest invited me to give a keynote address at a conference his team organized about the future of sport. They wanted to hear about current best practices for quantifying physical and mental health, and asked me to speculate about opportunities technology might provide sports with in the coming years. The Dean asked how technology would transform the future of sport at the end of our meeting before the conference. As a sports enthusiast, I spent a lot of time thinking about the future–how the lives of athletes, coaches, and spectators will change in response to technology.

Technology has been a major influence in athletics for decades. Professional timer services have changed Formula–1, cycling, swimming, or athletics by making every thousandth of a second count. The hawk–eye technique has helped track the trajectory of balls in cricket since 2001 and in tennis since 2004. In the video replay, we can clearly see whether the ball was in or out as the technique shows the whole route of it.

The performance of football players has been measured and assessed by a method introduced by UEFA in 2007. Sixteen cameras monitor the field so that officials can know accurately the trajectories of the players and the ball. They know what distance a player covered or how many passes he had. Goal–line technology assists ice hockey and football referees in deciding whether the ball was in or out. In American football referees can re–watch a play when the call is close. In basketball the NBA uses replay vision to review last–touch decisions in the final two minutes of the game.

The question is not whether technology can improve gamesmanship or the spectator experience but to what extent we will let it dominate. It started with simple fitness gadgets and GPS devices that measured distance and number of steps. But the range of opportunities is now enormous. Many athletes in professional clubs wear special shirts that measure their vital signs during practice or even games. Staff and players can make the best decisions about form and physical improvements.

For just this reason smart clothes have improved markedly in recent years. HexoSkin developed a shirt with sensors woven into it that measure heart rate, breathing, number of steps, pace, and calories burnt. The shirts are available in adult and junior sizes, and are marketed to professional athletes, researchers, and people who simply want to live more healthily. Currently battery life is less than a day, and you still need to attach a device to the shirt in order to measure your vital signs. Cirque de Soleil uses it to monitor performers' fatigue, for example. OMSignal offers similar shirts less expensively. Journalists who have tested them say it is probably worth waiting for the next generation. The shirts are not yet ready for mainstream use, although they show promise.

MC10 makes microchips that can measure numerous vital signs simultaneously. A biostamp chip called Checklight was added to a skullcap so it could detect if an athlete sustained a head injury after a collision. In another application, the biostamp could be stuck to a premature baby's skin in order to monitor body temperature constantly.

Two driving forces behind developing sports technology are improving athleticism and making more money. For decades doping has been problematic in cycling, baseball, and wrestling, among others. The future may have to contend with a different kind of doping, technological one.

An athlete can outperform others by either talent, lucky genetics, or good coaching. In jackpot situations, all these work, but good quality data are needed no matter the background. The better the microchips you use are and the better the data analysis is, the more promising the results will be. Athletes today can measure many parameters. For rowing, a company called Motionize developed an application that calculates everything from stroke length and heart rate to distance and distance per stroke. Another device, Skulpt, determines body fat percentage and muscle mass to optimize them to personalized training routines. The ShotTracker analyzes a player's baseball shots and suggests ways to improve technique.

With these devices athletes can play safer and train harder, and the whole process is automatically quantified. A weightlifter can train hard and do his best in competitions. Or he can measure every element of training, optimize his diet, and see how to get the most out of his genetic background in order to master the best form in competitions. It is clear that more athletes will turn towards disruptive innovations that can make them better and measure their progress.

The experience of exercise should change in amateur sports as well. With more comfortable and cheaper gadgets, measuring data will be seamless and easy for those who want to move just for fun. An app called Playpass lets people organize recreational leagues in many sports, and the app helps find participants. Other apps such as Sport42, Sportpartner, and BuddyUp help find people users can run or play football with. Social motivation can now play an important role in making people exercise more.

Devices and digital services are only a beginning. When assessing blood markers becomes widely available through retail services, athletes can start measuring the biological impact of their training routine. Now it is possible but complicated to do so. In a few years it will be as simple as taking one's pulse. The more biotechnology services an athlete has access to, the more likely they will optimize their form.

In addition to biomarkers, athletes can also find out how their particular genes contribute to performance. With this information they can personalize their training instead of following the routines that all players do. A company called Athletigen offers direct–to–consumer genetic testing and claims to compare one's scores to people around the world. The consumer sends in a saliva sample, and receives scores about motivation, endurance, recovery, injury protection, and anaerobic capacity.

Chinese scientists were rumored to be creating human embryos with specific genetic traits such as genes for athletic ability. There are no international standards about how one would do this safely and legally, and still many groups are trying to make genetically modified human embryos. Such an approach, even if true, would certainly fail because human characteristics are much more complicated and relay on far more than single genes.

Coaching will improve too and become more technologically rooted. Many football coaches film trainings with overhead cameras so that they can analyze how their players move before a big game. The method is simple compared to what companies such as ChryonHego, Catapult, and Kinexon offer. 3D motion tracking and smart analytics yield more precise data on each player. Each player is assigned quantifiable performance indicators the same way one assigns them in video games such as the FIFA football series or the NFL series in American football.

The spectator's perspective will change as well. First V1sion offers an integrated camera system attached to a player's uniform. This lets fans watch the game from the player's' point of view, and even switch the view from player to player. Many people might be willing to pay to see a football match from the perspective of Lionel Messi or Andres Iniesta. Iniesta has even backed the idea. The introduction of 3D and virtual reality devices will let fans see what Messi is experiencing out on the pitch. We will choose from what angle we want to watch the game and which player we are interested in.

US Major League Baseball had over 74 million in–stadium viewers in 2013. Events such as the Olympic Games, football World Cup finals, and the American Superbowl command more than 1 billion viewers through television and online channels. And we all watch the same screen. Imagine how it will change when the viewer experience becomes truly personalized. You get to be the director of your own sports programs.

Technology will transform whole areas of sport. Already, the first cyborg Olympic game will take place in Zurich in October 2016. Only people augmented by technology can enter to compete. I will definitely be there to witness this momentous event. As someone who has pursued different kinds of sports from football and squash to running and athletics, I look forward to improving my performance with data, although I don't want to let technology dominate my enjoyment of the beauty of sport.

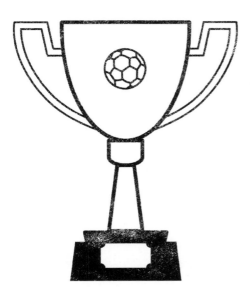
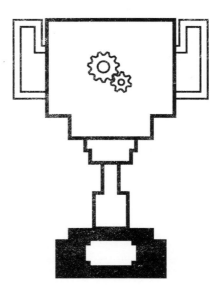

CHAPTER 2. DISRUPTIVE TRENDS

CAN ARTIFICIAL FOOD PUT AN END TO FAMINE?

#nutrition #canutr #DietaryGuidelines #healthchat I Soylent Green (1973)

I gave a keynote address at the 2014 Congress of the American Society for Clinical Pathology in Florida. They asked me to focus on the future of genomics and biotechnology given than many of their members work in these fields. I gave examples of genome sequencing, ways to design new drugs with microorganisms, and I mentioned how organs or food can be created now in laboratories. During the Presidential dinner that evening I chatted with a pathologist from Central Africa who asked me whether artificial food could put an end to famine. His country was suffering from food shortages and he wanted to know if fake food could be a solution.

The World Food Programme has some disheartening statistics about famine worldwide. About 805 million people don't have adequate nutrition. It means one in nine people globally. The highest percentage of undernourished populations is in Sub–Saharan Africa. Poor nutrition causes nearly half the deaths in children under five years–old. About 66 million schoolchildren across the world are hungry. The list goes on. Ensuring food security and receiving relief from other countries could drive these numbers lower than they were in the 1990s when over a billion people were undernourished. But there is still a lot to do. Given that traditional approaches haven't mitigated the problem satisfactorily, we might ask what technology can offer.

Producing food today is incredibly stressful to the environment. About one third of what we produce goes to waste. Imagine any other enterprise working that ineffectively. And that waste contains ingredients it's increasingly hard to collect. As sensor cost goes down and automation efficiency goes up, robots will gradually replace farm workers.

Actually, robotic examples are already at hand. The WP5 robot can autonomously harvest peppers grown in a greenhouse. It is self–propelled, and has a camera and lighting. Such a robot will be economically viable when it can pick a fruit or vegetable every six seconds, costs less than $220,000, and lasts for at least 5 years. Some farmers use self–driving tractors that guide themselves via radar instead of using topological maps and GPS. Drones can monitor large areas and detect irrigation problems. Their resolution is higher than that of satellites, and they are cheaper to use than airplanes. A wine–bot can keep an eye on vineyard health and check the soil. It can navigate around plant nurseries, and move potted seedlings according to a touchscreen plan made by humans. While there will always be tasks that only people can perform, the cost and efficiency of farming should respectively decrease and increase.

As farming becomes more technological, agriculture is turning its attention to artificial food. The Cultured Beef Project aims to create artificial meat in the laboratory. Technicians remove muscle cells from the shoulder of a cow, and feed the cells with a nutrient mix in a Petri dish, and they grow into muscle tissue. From a few starter cells one can derive tens of tons of meat. The whole world could be fed with meat from muscle cells grown in a lab.

In 2013 the cost of lab–grown meat for a hamburger was $325,000. By 2015 it had dropped to $11. The biggest obstacle so far is not technology but the taste–that is unlike what people are used to because blood, fat, and connective tissue are missing. But researchers are working to improve that. The slogan of a similar company, Modern Meadow, says that the "future is cultured, not slaughtered".

A team in San Francisco is working on vegan cheese that contains protein identical to milk protein but doesn't come from animals. They transform yeast cells into miniature milk–protein factories. It isn't a cheese substitute, but real cheese that has no animal origin. Their process is more environmentally sustainable than standard cheese–making.

For eight thousand years we have been collecting and drinking animal milk. Nowadays, the environmental and economic costs of producing milk are huge, and so animal–free milk would be welcome. The startup Muufri hopes to design yeast cultures that can produce milk proteins. This retains the taste and nutritional value of real milk. It could be accessible to many people worldwide less expensively than dairy milk. Dairy production is responsible for about 3% of global greenhouse gas emissions every year. Muufri argues that making an entire cow to make just the milk is inefficient. They can control what the milk actually contains, and while their milk cannot provide the same quality that Mother Nature does, it can come close. We will see whether regulatory authorities will agree.

Elon Musk once told the daughter of an advisor: „If there was a way I could not eat so I could work more, I would not eat. I wish there was a way to get nutrients without sitting down for a meal." The company Soylent is working on it. A meal replacement powder that contains all the nutrition required by an average adult is mixed with water. The company advises consumers to supplement traditional meals until they find their preferred balance between Soylent and real food. The company hopes its product will save time and effort by eliminating the need to prepare every meal. The cost is around $3 per meal. As of 2015, it has been "generally recognized as safe" by the FDA, but no one has yet produced any data about the risks or the potential benefits.

Eventually people may start printing out food at home. Those who want to turn to technological solutions instead of spending time with preparing and cooking meals will have a chance to use 3D printers at home.

The Foodini project received great attention when the first articles were published about printing out food at home. CMO & Co–founder of Natural Machines, Lynette Kucsma told me the plan is to print food using fresh ingredients instead of creating artificial food. Even her first reaction was negative about the concept of printing out food. But a device connected to the Internet and controlled via touchscreen devices can lead to better understanding and reproducing family recipes for generations. There are no food capsules in the machine called Foodini, but the software makes it easy to print recipes and users can make their own recipes.

Currently Foodini can print out sweets, meals, snacks, cookies, chocolates, crackers, breadsticks, spaghettis, burgers, and even ready–to–bake pizza. An online community shares what members come up with. Such devices would like to be considered kitchen appliances. We preload the food in the device in the morning where it stays fresh. Before leaving for home, we send a notification through a smartphone app to the device, and the meal is going to get ready by the time we get home. Although Foodini currently focuses more on customized food design mostly for pastries instead of cooking a meal.

In two generations there may be no one left who knows how to cook. We will print what we need in the way depicted in movies such as *The Fifth Element* or *Back to the Future II*. Kucsma believes that the opposite should take place. Fresh ingredients must be prepared and we have to know what is in our food. Food scanners could be of help in this. In the future, specialty supermarkets could become available that would make the process simpler with ready–to–print products. Technology is about making our lives easier, not how to change the way we eat. As Kucsma says, the test is in the taste.

A 2015 Kickstarter scheme called Bocusini strove to print out precision objects in sugar and marzipan. A simple 3D printer with a heated extrusion head uses cartridges of marzipan, chocolate, and fudge. The German team behind the idea wants people to be able to hack this food printer to make it personalized and use it at home from 2016.

Biozoon prints out gourmet-looking food for seniors who need to eat purified meals. ZMorph and Choc Edge can print out chocolate in whatever forms the user wants. In 2013, NASA's food printer has printed a proof-of-concept thin pizza that baked in 70 seconds after printing. Such a printer could provide Mars colonizers with all the vitamins and minerals they need. And the end product is not always pizza, but anything they can model through the software.

All these methods have to be in compliance with current, and yet not even existing regulations, but let's be honest. We are not going to feed billions of people who have growing needs without turning to disruptive technologies. We need a healthy attitude and rules that help innovators ease the lives of more than 800 million worldwide, and still it doesn't take out the joy from eating delicious meals.

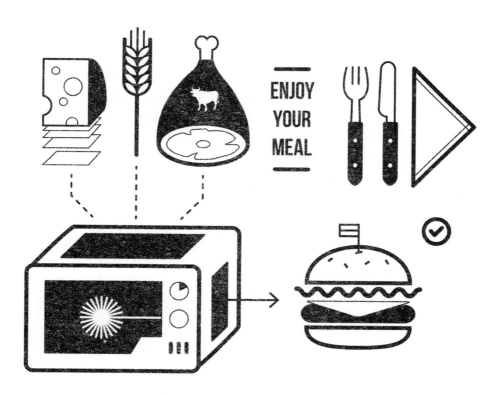

WHAT COMES AFTER THE WEARABLE REVOLUTION?

#wearables #wearabletech #medicalfuture | Total Recall (1990)
Johnny Mnemonic (1995)

An investor forum on the US east coast invited me to talk about an exciting question: what comes after the wearable revolution? When I spoke, I demonstrated all the devices and methods I use to measure my health parameters. I then described what I think could come when wearables penetrate the mainstream.

A growing population is already using wearable devices. The market will continue to grow while devices will shrink in size, get cheaper, and be more comfortable. At present it is essentially impossible to over–track one's health. It's the first time in history we've been able to do it digitally. By the time tracking technology gets better we should have arrived at a stage when we know what to measure, why and how.

But it seems other technology besides wearables will be ready simultaneously. In many cases, smart clothes are merely traditional garments with a few sensors. Genuinely smart fabrics will be able to communicate, transform, and change color based on the wearer's mood.

Special fabrics might enhance performance by regulating body temperature, reducing wind resistance, or controlling muscle vibration, the principal cause of muscle fatigue. A company called CuteCircuit had a fashion show in New York in which models controlled the appearance of their dresses via smartphones. Fundawear is a wearable technology that allows physical touch to be transferred from a smartphone app to a partner anywhere in the world. Couples wearing Fundawear can tickle each other from a distance as the points where they touch their own T–shirt are activated in the T–shirt of the partner. The world of fashion is poised to embrace wearable technology.

To accomplish this, extremely thin electronics are needed. Such e–textiles or fibretronics have electronic properties. Sometimes such fibretronics are called digital tattoos. For example, VivaLNK has a small adhesive near–field communication (NFC) tag that sticks to the skin. It is water–proof and lasts for five days. Wearer's phone is unlocked by moving it close to the tattoo. It can also activate the camera, access Twitter, and compose an e–mail. Yet it is still wearable technology.

A microchip could be attached to the skin and measure any health parameters. When there is something the wearer should take care of, it sends a notification to the smartphone or smartwatch. The group of Professor Takao Someya in Japan is dedicated to developing the thinnest sensors that measures everything we need. In 2015, they released a wearable and printable temperature sensor that can remotely notify of fever. Probably the fashion industry will bring this technology closer to people than medical applications.

Another class of tools could be called digestibles because they are capsules or tiny gadgets that one swallows. AdhereTech designed a smart wireless pill box. It notifies patients by phone or text message when they miss their medication. It could improve patient compliance or monitor drug absorption. Colonoscopy is not the most comfortable medical procedure, but it is often a necessary one. Given Imaging's PillCam is a standard–size capsule with a camera inside that can be easily swallowed and visualizes the digestive system.

Proteus Health has developed pills that contain a sensor the size of a sand grain. When the pill reaches the stomach it signals a patch worn by the patient that confirms the medication has been taken. Patients receive updates on a smartphone, and set medication reminders, while their caregivers can access the data on a web portal to learn about the efficacy of the treatment. For the first time, taking a medication becomes a controllable and detectable process. Big data can help make better decisions which have not been available before such pills with sensors.

So–called insideables will be implanted inside the body or just under the skin. Already some people have radio–frequency identification (RFID) implants with which they can open up a laptop, control a smartphone, or operate a garage door. RFID tags have been used in industries from transportation to animal tracking. The US Department of Veterans Affairs announced plans to use RFIDs in hospitals to improve care and reduce costs. This way, patients could be easily recognized by walking through a door with a sensor instead of using expensive and slow methods.

The first RFID chips were allowed to be implanted into people in 2004 by the FDA. The FDA has taken steps such as working with manufacturers and the RFID industry to inform the public about its potential effects on medical devices. Having chips implanted may sound like dystopian science fiction, but a Swedish company actually asked its employees to do this in 2015. The chips let open security doors, use the copy machine, or pay for their lunch without needing credit cards or pin codes. Not all employees were thrilled by the idea.

Amal Graafstra, author of RFID Toys was one of the first people to get an implanted chip. A cosmetic surgeon used a scalpel to place a microchip in his left hand, and his family doctor injected a chip into his right hand. He launched Dangerous Things, which sells anyone RFIDs, and finds either tattoo artists or doctors to surgically implant them. This practice is questionable. As public interest grows, oversight and regulations should get stricter for the sake of patient safety.

Currently, the ethical and privacy issues outweigh any conceivable benefits that the technology might provide. Until we have more experience and better oversight, we can only witness the evolution of wearables–tattoos–digestibles–insideables.

We will have to adjust our vocabulary to a new wearable slang. For example, jerktech makes people antisocial. Hearables are ear computers. Nearables only work when a smartphone is nearby. Awareables sense their surroundings, and thereables are present in the spaces we move through during the day. Google recently formed a partnership with Levis to create smart textiles. The fashion world will be adding new terms to this glossary soon.

Whether I wear, digest or implant it, I enjoy learning more about how I respond to medications; how fast I digest them; and how these all help me make better decisions about my life.

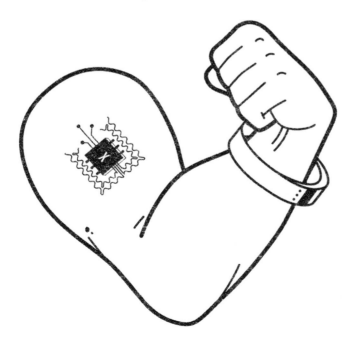

WILL WE 3D PRINT OR GROW ORGANS?

#3dprinting #biotech | The Island (2005) Splice (2009)

I accept invitations to give presentations available to the general public because it is one of the most efficient methods for disseminating information about the future of medicine. After a talk I gave in Bilbao, Spain a woman asked about either printing or growing human organs in the future. She was not particularly interested in the technology, but she has lost her father for lack of organ donors. He needed a new kidney due to a chronic illness and the transplantation waiting list was long. Was there hope for the hundreds of thousands of people who are waiting for a suitable organ?

She made an important point. In the US alone, on average eighteen people die every day from the lack of available organs. Every 14 minutes someone is added to a kidney transplant list. How brutal is it that a patient who needs an organ transplant either has to wait for someone to donate it while alive or die?

The first transplant took place in 1905 when a cornea from an injured 11–year–old boy was transplanted into the eye of a 45–year–old farmer who had damaged one of his eyes in an accident. During World War I skin grafts were implanted on British soldiers. Transplantation of a major organ took place in 1954 when a 23–year–old from Massachusetts donated one of his kidneys to his twin who suffered from chronic nephritis.

Technology exists that assists organs in doing their function instead of having to replace them. Impella is the smallest heart pump in use today. It is the size of a pencil and is FDA approved to support the heart for up to six hours during cardiac surgeries. HeartMate II will act like a pair of cardiac crutches. It is the size of an avocado, and people have been living with it for years. All the recipients have an almost undetectable pulse. When those hearts have to be replaced in the future one hopes that tissue engineering will have matured.

I had a quick chat with Dr. Anthony Atala, director of Wake Forest's Institute for Regenerative Medicine, one of the most progressive places when it comes to tissue regeneration. His team developed the first lab–grown organ: a bladder that was implanted in a real person. He still practices urology to learn more about patient needs. Certain tissues, he said, such as blood vessels, vagina, and urine tubes, have already been grown in the lab and implanted in a small number of patients undergoing clinical trials. Scientists around the world are working to expand the number of tissues that can be engineered and the number of patients who might benefit from them. The most difficult organs to engineer are the heart, liver, kidney, and pancreas. Many patients die while waiting to receive one.

Professor Atala thinks the future of bioprinting could look like the Dell model. Your surgeon ships your tissue sample to a company. A few days later, the organ arrives in a sterile container via FedEx, ready for implantation. Think of it as a piece of me made to order. He emphasized that there are no surgical challenges, only technological ones. If we can overcome those hurdles then engineered tissue can function like the original one.

He believes scientists will one day successfully restore function to damaged, complex organs, either through cell therapies or perhaps by inserting a slice of functioning engineered tissue into the damaged organ. It will take many years of endeavor to come about. It is not something we can expect in the immediate future. We are far away from printing organs on demand. Holding out false hope should be avoided.

There are exceptions such as the company Organovo. They are actively developing a line of human tissues for use in medical research and drug discovery. These include both normal tissues and specially designed disease models. They are also working on the development of specific tissues for use in clinical patient care.

In 2014 they announced the successful printing of liver tissue that functioned like a real liver for weeks. The three–dimensional liver models, known as exVive3D, are only a few millimeters wide. One print head of the 3D bioprinter deposits a support matrix. The other head precisely places human liver cells in it. The tissue contains all cell types normally found in the liver. It can produce proteins such as albumin and fibrinogen, and also synthesize cholesterol. Previous models were two–dimensional. The 3D version can distinguish between toxic and harmless compounds. The long–term goal is to eliminate animal testing by pharmaceutical companies given that such liver tissues could assess the toxicity of potential drugs.

Another astonishing demonstration occurred at the Experimental Biology conference in April 2015. Fully functional human kidney tubular tissues had been generated with Organovo's 3D bioprinter. Given that 80% of patients waiting for organ donors are waiting for a kidney, this development could show the general public that bioprinting is not merely a promise. After this, even sci–fi lovers will find it hard to imagine what comes next.

Biomaterials are both printed out and grown in glassware. In 2014, cells that developed into a thymus, an organ that helps fight infections, were transplanted into thymus–depleted mice. Researchers had reprogrammed embryo cells of the mice to develop into immune cells. Since then bladders, urethras, and windpipes have been grown in the labs.

The recipe looks simple but is quite a feat. They scan the patient's organ to determine personalized size and shape. Then they create a scaffold to give cells something to grow on in three dimensions. They then add cells from the patient to this scaffold. Finally, a bioreactor creates the optimal environment for the cells to grow into an organ. Cells are actually very picky, and it is quite difficult to grow them the way one wants—or even have them grow at all. But eventually, researchers find ways to make it happen.

Synthetic skin, a bionic ear, bladder, or cornea might be the first organs to be either bioprinted or grown in the lab on demand. After that, more complicated ones might be engineered to be fully functioning organs. Twenty years from now we might look back at transplantation waiting lists and marvel at what a brutal world it was in 2015.

I don't like to ruin this optimistic and positive vision of the future, but if regulations are not sufficiently strict and clear, the black market for printed organs will thrive. As soon as scaffolds are available and methods are open source, people around the world will be tempted to start printing unregulated and untested biomaterials, and sell them to desperate people.

Another scenario is asking for new organs only because they can afford them. Instead of changing lifestyle or stopping habits such as smoking or drinking, they might rather buy a new organ. This will be a knotty ethical issue.

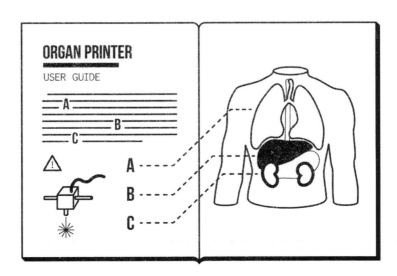

ORGAN PRINTER
USER GUIDE

CAN PARALYZED PEOPLE EVER WALK AGAIN?

#exoskeleton | The Matrix Reloaded (2003) Avatar (2009)

Some of the questions I have received over the years have been very emotional. If a talk is engaging and the audience is open–minded, people tend to ask highly personal questions. Once I was asked to speak about augmentation–what would happen if we augmented our human capabilities simply because we can? I spoke about brain implants, robotic prosthetics, and powered exoskeletons. A woman in a wheelchair was the first to pose a question. She told her story about the accident she had years ago and how different her life was in the wheelchair. She wanted to know whether paralyzed people can walk ever again.

She was not alone in her predicament. An estimated 12,500 people sustain spinal cord injuries every year. As of 2014, 300,000 individuals in the US alone were living with such injuries.

Although ongoing technological developments make me an optimist, I have to answer such questions with care. A given technology might be available, but not affordable for everyone. Or a technology may exist, but cannot fully restore function. In this woman's case I could be optimistic and realistic at the same time. Yes, paralyzed people will be able to walk again. Even the sense of touch may be restored. Eventually prosthetics may be controlled with one's thoughts.

In my talk I described the story of Amanda Boxtel who got paralyzed from the waist down following a skiing accident. After she started her new life in a wheelchair she joined an expedition to Antarctica, carried an Olympic torch, and kept on working to change her life. When she started working with Ekso Bionics, a company in California, she became hopeful.

A few years later, I watched her stand up from her wheelchair and walk around thanks to a backpack computer that powered her exoskeleton. A robotic structure attached to her joints and supplied enough muscle power to enable her to walk. It was actually a wearable robot. Thousands of patients have been learning to walk again thanks to their exoskeleton.

I asked Russ Angold, chief technology officer, how the company imagined the future. He said they saw a day when people who previously couldn't walk because of paralysis or other forms of leg weakness regain the ability. Whether exoskeletons will assist them entirely, providing power to their legs when the individuals cannot, or whether because of other medical breakthroughs; exoskeletons will continue to play a role in human augmentation.

The use of exoskeletons is expanding into other industries. A passive industrial product, Ekso Works, augments an individual who works with heavy equipment. This could be an effective tool to reduce load weight and potential injuries while increasing efficiency at the same time. With further refinements and cost–efficient 3D printing, powered exoskeletons may eventually be more like clothing and less like the clunky exoskeletons of today.

Another device is ReWalk, designed in Israel and priced at $85,000 as of 2015. The company garnered major attention when the FDA approved its use in US hospitals in 2011, and again when the FDA approved its use in the home and in public in 2014. Dozens of devices are scheduled to become commercially available 2016.

Such exoskeletons could be used in emergency situations such as fires and earthquakes. Lifting huge weights and walking around without becoming fatigued and avoiding injury would be a great asset to emergency workers. An exoskeleton boot released in April 2015 reduced the fatigue caused by walking by 7%. The device is lighter than powered devices, weighing about half a kilogram, and the performance boost is notable.

Unsurprisingly, armies around the world want to develop combat exoskeletons for their soldiers. DARPA is funding the Warrior Web project, which is developing an exoskeleton that soldiers can wear under their clothing and which will help them run faster, climb more easily, and jump higher than they typically can. The design will lighten physical loads, lessen injuries, and augment muscular power.

Walking and jumping are not enough. The real challenge is letting paralyzed individuals feel again when their robot arm touches something. Amazing as they are, it is not easy to walk with exoskeletons or use robotic prosthetics. Learning to do so takes time, and is made more difficult by the lack of tactile feedback, the ability to feel when the foot touches the floor or the hand touches a surface. Sensor–laden prosthetics let patients adapt to variations in walking speed and environmental conditions.

Electronic skins being developed now let patients to even feel pressure via their prosthetics. Think about it for a moment in sci–fi terms. The end goal of all prosthetics and exoskeletons is to restore human function. That implies that prosthetic devices should be controllable by the user's thoughts. While there have been improvements in neuroprosthetics, robotic movements tended to be jerky, and the thought control wasn't really intuitive. Users had to think through the movements they wanted to make step by step. Newer iterations let patients control robotic arms by intention alone. One patient with such a device could shake hands, drink from a cup, and play rock–paper–scissors.

That patient is Erik Sorto, who was paralyzed after a gunshot wound to his neck. He received a microchip implant into the part of his brain that is responsible for planning and imagining activities. He can now move his robotic arm by mere thought. Researchers plan to implant a second chip in a sensory part of his brain. That way, when the robot touches something it will signal to the patient's brain and let him feel what the robot feels.

By 2030 exoskeletons and related neuroprosthetic devices may be so thin and affordable that paralysis would no longer be a health issue. Research is so promising that soon the biggest issue may be over–augmentation. People might want to get paralyzed or damage a limb in order to get a robotic one. They might think as such technologies can give them more strength and power, they are more beneficial than their wholesome body parts. When prosthetics become sophisticated and advanced at an affordable price, this will become a public issue.

People who aren't paralyzed might nonetheless want to jump higher or not get fatigued when walking for miles. What will be the threshold for using this technology? How will doctors respond when patients demand new robotic arms? What will society do if people will not want to move around anymore because sitting and transporting in an exoskeleton is easier? These questions demonstrate some of the challenges we will face by the time the most important ones have been solved and when formerly paralyzed people can walk faster than the rest of us.

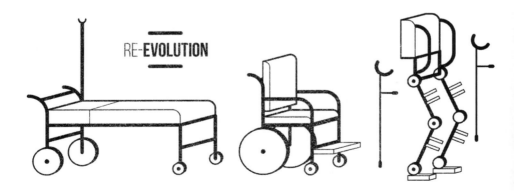

RE-EVOLUTION

SHOULD I GET MY GENOME SEQUENCED?

#genomics #medicalfuture #NGS | The 6th Day (2000)

My childhood dream was to become a genetics researcher. When I reached this goal at the age of 26, I decided to create a new profession in which my geek self was also involved. This is how I became a medical futurist. But genetics has still been close to my heart, and so I'm glad whenever I am invited to speak about my experience with genetic testing.

Direct–to–consumer genetic testing was a big thing in the early 2010s. New companies offering such services appeared month after month. I have used three such services, and I like to share what they provided me with, and how, as a geneticist, I analyzed my own DNA information.

After one talk I gave about this a woman in her early twenties told me how worried she was that many types of cancer had affected her family. Given the examples I had described she wanted to know whether she should have her genome sequenced. She was curious whether doing so could tell her what to expect in the coming years. She believed that having information about our DNA comes with a verdict. But it does not.

I had my own DNA analyzed while doing my PhD, which made the process quite an adventure. Companies sent me sampling tubes that I sent back with my saliva containing cells and DNA. A few weeks later I could browse my ancestry and see which famous people I share a genetic background with. But the trick part was seeing what medical conditions I had a predetermined risk for.

Tens of thousands of studies have analyzed the connections between genetic codes and specific diseases. If you have cytosine instead of guanine at a certain position in your DNA, you have a bigger risk for developing asthma. Genetic testing companies design their own algorithms and choose what studies to use while calculating your disease risk. For the same DNA sample I received three different results for the same conditions. One company told me I have an elevated risk for diabetes. Another one said that my risk is lower than the general population's. I had to be a geneticist in order to draw any conclusions from these.

Actions that could actually make a difference to me were missing. I would have liked to learn what lifestyle changes could decrease my risk for developing the conditions each company mentioned. But the same advice popped up from all of them for each condition: have a healthy diet, exercise more, don't smoke, and don't drink alcohol to excess. Oh yes, and have a check up from your physician once in a while.

I got fed up with inconsistent results, and decided to analyze the genome myself. I downloaded the raw data of my DNA into a huge text file containing codes that seemed to make no sense, and uploaded it to a service called Promethease. It costs $5 to do so. But the analysis it provides doesn't tell you what to think. Instead, it lets you discover associations between your DNA and known diseases. In seconds, a huge list appeared on my monitor showing me the highest correlations between my DNA and the findings of numerous studies. I started browsing and immediately learned interesting things.

It marked findings as good or positive, such as my ability to taste bitterness, my decreased risk for autism, Crohn's disease, colorectal and lung cancer, and my resistance to Prion disease (the kind of infectious particles that cause mad–cow disease). It marked findings as bad or negative, such as a less robust serotonin processing that can make me susceptible to novelty seeking (which my job depends on), an increased risk for type–2 diabetes, insulin resistance, and nicotine dependence. To be clear, the same conditions appeared on both lists many times. It is hard to draw final conclusions given this. But it was enjoyable to learn my muscle performance is consistent with being a sprinter. It explains why I've been one since the age of 6, and why I hate running for long distances.

Analyzing genetic information should be much smoother and more efficient than it is now. I see sequencing my DNA soon costing less than shipping the sample. Billions of genomes will be available before we can practically use the information in medical decision–making. Genome sequencing will also become a storage issue, making informatics a bottleneck.

In 2013 the FDA published its concerns about what direct–to–consumer services really provide. It also questioned the scientific background behind them. Their scrutiny led to shutting down most of the mail–order services, leaving genetic testing in the purview of institutions and medical professionals. After its initial hype, direct–to–consumer genomics is plummeting. Soon I think they will rise again like the phoenix.

When Illumina, a company offering sequencing services, announced in 2014 that hundreds of thousands of new genomes would become available soon, it was a signal that the price per sequencing would be under $1,000. As the price continues to go down, the number of people wanting their genomes sequenced will skyrocket. It should reach a million around 2017, and ten million by 2020.

Services will be available for newborns that provide parents with their sequence data. This can even be done prenatally, because the child's DNA can be extracted from the mother's blood. This can tell parents what illnesses their child will face during their lifetime.

All of this leads us to genetic engineering. When we can make diagnoses based on genetic backgrounds? What will prevent people from making changes to their genomes when the method to do so becomes available? Gene therapies exist for Parkinson's disease, certain immune conditions, and a form of leukemia. The first gene therapy treatment was approved only in 2012.

In April of 2015, Chinese researchers reported that they could edit the DNA of non–viable embryos. This launched major ethical debates. The problem lies not in wanting to cure diseases this way, but when this impulse turns to enhancing existing capabilities rather than repairing damaged ones. Transhumanists could talk about this for hours.

When devices capable of DNA sequencing become small enough and simple to use they might be employed in the home. Oxford NanoPore's MinION is a portable device for real–time analysis of DNA. Samples include blood, serum, or water. It connects to a computer through USB and can analyze immediately. DNA sequencing today takes place in huge institutions with rows of machines working tirelessly. Then an army of bioinformatics experts makes the data available. If portable devices reach a certain efficiency and quality, cognitive computers could do the hard job of transforming the pure data into conclusions relevant to everyday health.

Newer services such as uBiome go even further. It offers genome sequencing of the bacteria that live in our digestive system. By analyzing the composition of these organisms, it can tell customers whether they have the microbiome of heavy drinkers, vegetarians, or athletes. While individuals can obtain the sequence of their DNA and that of their gut bacteria, making medical decisions based on that information is fraught.

The biggest issues in the coming years will be the cost of sequencing dropping to almost zero, and the improvement in quality of conclusions that are drawn from the data as well as the general understanding of what genomics can provide. It is worth having our DNA data, but it might be worth waiting a little bit longer.

A genome is not about predestination, but risks. Genetics loads the gun, lifestyle pulls the trigger. Unless we become experts about our own health, even the most detailed genetic report will be useless.

AGCTGACTCTAGTG
ACGCTAGTACAGCG
TACTAGTCTGACGC
TAGTACAGCTAGTC
CATGATGCTCGAGT
ACAGCTGACTCTAG

WILL THE MEDICAL TRICORDER FROM STAR TREK BECOME REAL?

#wearabletech #digitalhealth #tricorder #mhealth | Cloud Atlas (2012)

As a movie fan, I love talking about how the science fiction movies of the last hundred years have shaped our ideas about medical technology. When university students doing film studies asked me to give a talk, I was thrilled. I divided the history of science fiction into five eras and came up with movie examples for each. I demonstrated what technologies those movies and television series inspired, and what others they stole from real life. I dedicated a whole section to technology that *Star Trek* inspired. The long list included telepresence, the hypospray for painless injections, the voice–activated communicator, the iPad, diagnostic beds that tracked numerous vital signs, and of course the famous medical tricorder.

When Dr McCoy grabbed his tricorder and scanned a patient, the portable, hand–held device immediately listed vital signs, other parameters, and a diagnosis. It was the Swiss Army knife for physicians. When our class discussion turned to potential medical uses, a doubtful student asked how such a thing could work in real when it came from science fiction. I then gave him another list to consider. A visual display device from *Star Trek* is Google Glass now. The heads–up display in *Minority Report* is air touch technology. *Iron Man* is currently being developed by DARPA. The self–directed vacuum cleaner from *The Jetsons* now exists as Roomba. I could go on.

A working tricorder could bring about a new era in medicine. Instead of expensive machines and long waiting times, information would be available immediately. Physicians could scan a patient, or patients could scan themselves and receive a list of diagnostic options and suggestions. Imagine the influence it could have on underdeveloped regions. It should not substitute for medical supervision, but when there is none it comes in handy.

It could be useful when a diagnosis needs confirming or when standard laboratory equipment is not available. A high–power microscope with a smartphone, for example, could analyze swab samples and photos of skin lesions. Sensors could pick up abnormalities in DNA, or detect antibodies and specific proteins. An electronic nose, an ultrasonic probe, or almost anything we have now could be yoked to a smartphone and augment its features.

An in–person doctor visit includes assessing the patient's condition, health parameters, and other data. Much of this could be performed without needing the presence of a medical professional. I'm merely pointing out an absence of medical staff is the case in many regions of the world.

This situation is an impetus behind the Nokia Sensing X Challenge that has called for teams to design prototypes of a working tricorder. It should measure a wide range of biomarkers with a dropplet of blood, be able to diagnose malaria, high blood pressure, and similar conditions, as well as monitor epilepsy. The winning finalist teams are expected to test their prototypes with thousands of users in 2015.

The Qualcomm Tricorder X Prize was announced in 2012 to motivate innovators in this direction. It featured 230 teams from thirty countries, and promised an award of $10 million to the first team to build a working medical tricorder. The device had to correctly diagnose fifteen different medical conditions from a sore throat to sleep apnea and colon cancer.

Using these devices should also be intuitive so that anyone who understands a smartphone should be able to operate them. Consumer usability is almost as important as medical accuracy. A friendly interface will count when choosing a winner. Teams from Northern Ireland, the US, Slovenia, India, Taiwan, Canada, and the United Kingdom are working on systems that can analyze samples of blood, urine, and saliva.

I must warn that these competitions do not and cannot substitute for clinical trials. There are safety, privacy, legal, and liability issues that can only be assessed during strict trials.

The first working medical tricorder is the Scanadu Scout, a hand–held sensor held against a patient's forehead. It measures heart rate, breathing rate, blood oxygenation percentage, and body temperature. It can also take a reading of blood pressure, the electrocardiogram, and stress levels. The company is also working on Scanadu Urine for home use, which will give users data about liver, kidney, urinary tract, and metabolic functions. A smartphone app will guide users through the test procedure, process the test results, and explain them. This is also a big potential for error or human misinterpretation.

Viatom Technology in China released CheckMe in 2014. It measures ECG, pulse, oxygen saturation, blood pressure, body temperature, sleep quality, and daily activity. Vitaliti from CloudDx measures the same and sends data to the cloud. It lets users know about posture, physical activities and vital signs.

A big part of practicing medicine today is the way to obtain vital signs. The tricorder could bypass this problem by making vital signs and even lab markers immediately available either at home, at the doctor's office, or at remote locations that lack medical supervision. Today a doctor's expertise is needed to analyze as well as collect the data. The creativity and wisdom of physicians will be hard to get replaced. But obtaining data with a device should be something a 5 year–old could perform, and only technology can bring this to us. Empathy and a patient's emotions cannot be scanned, but vital signs can be.

It is possible that the FDA or other authorities will oppose the development of such a device, or that physicians will not be happy about patients getting the chance to do a health checkup themselves. They cannot stop this, but they could regulate the industry. The question is when we will start using medical tricorders, not whether we will use them. This is a good chance if we want people to access affordable care.

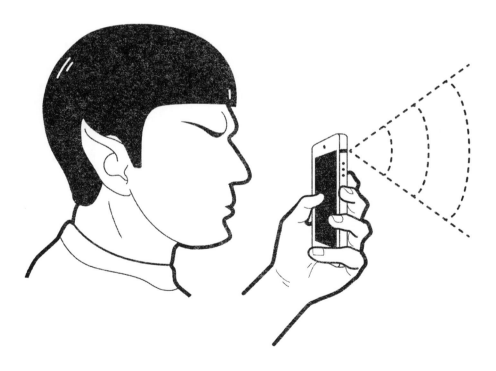

WHY ARE SUPERCOMPUTERS STILL NOT USED IN HEALTHCARE?

#ibmwatson #digitalhealth #supercomputer | Minority Report (2002)

In 2014 IBM invited me to speak at a local conference organized around big data. I was asked to discuss how supercomputers could assist physicians in the practice of medicine. After the talk an excited employee said he didn't see any reason why supercomputers weren't being used in healthcare. He thought it was only a matter of time.

At another event at the Hungarian Academy of Sciences I spoke about the future of big data in health. A professor of economics in his eighties stood up and asked his question in a sarcastic tone. He implied that if using supercomputers would make healthcare cheaper in the long term, then why we haven't been using them in massive quantities. The attitudes behind both questioners were different, but answer for each of them was the same.

Supercomputers have enormous speed and memory. They are used in weather forecasting, climate research, oil and gas exploration, or cracking encryption codes. Their capacity has been increasing according to Moore's law for decades. Most of them are in the US and China. Supercomputers can do 10^{15} calculations per second. If current trends hold, it will go up to 10^{18} by 2018. A machine that was considered a supercomputer in 1985 is now the equivalent of a smartwatch. This means a trillion–fold rise in computing power in less than 20 years.

For decades, we have been collecting data either in our own lives or in a healthcare setting. For decades, we have likewise struggled to do something with it. There are many ways that supercomputers could simplify and improve the lives of both physicians and patients. Patients spend a lot of time waiting for their doctors; doctors lose a lot of time waiting for a patient or a test result. A smart system could eliminate waiting times by scheduling people as efficiently as possible, directing them to the next logical place or task. Every day a doctor takes a lot of calls, in–person queries, e–mails, and messages from social media channels. In this torrent of information not every urgent matter can reach them. But a system could select the crucial ones out of the mess and direct the physician's attention to where it is actually needed.

It could prioritize e–mails, find needed information, keep users up–to–date about their treatment, perform administrative tasks, or make hard decisions rational. Imagine receiving all the pieces of information needed to make a particular decision including statistics, studies and collected wisdom concerning the patient's case in a digestible way. It could help physicians collaborate more easily, and would itself improve over time. Without super-computing power, healthcare will not improve or get cheaper.

Numerous cases have shown the advantages supercomputers offer in analyzing medical and health data. Using DNA found in the bones of a boy who died 24,000 years ago, a supercomputer in Texas compared his genetic background to that of modern people. A Silicon Valley company, Palantir, found the source of an E. coli outbreak and prevented further spread of contaminated products. MIT has predicted that by 2018 a global network of millions of genomes could be medicine's next great advance.

Imagine what medical conclusions could be drawn if all the genomes ever sequenced could be analyzed and compared to each other. What further associations between genetic background and health consequences could be discovered? We could then use all that information with readily available vital signs at our fingertips. Obviously, no layperson will be able to make medical decisions based on these, therefore help will be needed.

A patient gets a notification on their smartphone when they should get their health checked by a physician. An app could show me what influence my current lifestyle will have on my health as it has the data from other people with the same habits, age, gender, and vital signs. This is going to be easier to persuade people to live a healthy life. Or it might give them a false sense of security that they don't have to take care of themselves anymore. Solution lies somewhere between.

The Internet of things, the network of devices and apps connected to one another, has the potential to bring these analytical opportunities to life. It will provide physicians with checklists so they don't forget something important in medical decision–making. It will provide patients with everyday suggestions about how to live better lives. Data will help us decide what to eat based on our nutritional needs and genetic background. It will use all medical information from studies and devices used by patients to help make informed decisions only. Does that sound too optimistic? There is a reason it does.

If visions of prosperity cannot help bring this forward, cost efficiency will persuade hospital managers and policy makers to invest in supercomput-ers. A 2013 paper concluded that using an artificial intelligence algorithm not only decreased the overall cost of making a diagnosis compared to traditional methods; but also that the outcomes were better. Better informed decisions lead to lower healthcare costs.

I had a chat with Albert–László Barabási, the worldwide expert of network medicine who showed that there are hidden patterns behind everything from e–mails to daily habits. He thinks we can predict and uncover disease–disease relationships through the protein network, the so–called interactome which is incomplete at this time. He and his team think that behind each disease there are molecular fingerprints and hidden patterns which can only be described via smart algorithms and bioinformatic methods. They have been developing methods to interpret genetic data to drug target identification. It could begin to reclassify the relationships between diseases and their molecular background.

Before you think that most healthcare institutions cannot afford a supercomputer, consider that a professor and his 6 year–old son built one using only credit–card sized computers called Raspberry Pi, and Lego blocks. The computer cluster cost less than $4,000.

We can now start discovering the options supercomputers can give to us by feeding them with data that have already been around but from which we couldn't draw many conclusions. Cost and privacy will remain issues, but no system can be improved without first measuring data about it.

Imagine healthcare that has clear information about the effectiveness and success rates of its doctors and hospitals. Analyzing the data that pours into the system could tell us whether patients comply with their therapy. Would this be a breach of our private lives and the birth of the Big Brother? There is a chance for that, and this might be the price for living a healthy life and improving healthcare to its full potential. Unless someone comes up with a better idea or everyone becomes committed to living healthily.

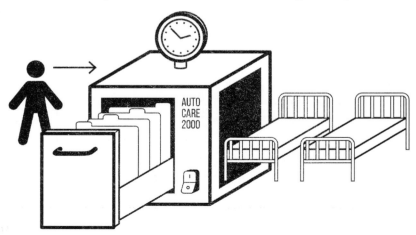

COULD DOCTORS LITERALLY LOOK THROUGH PATIENTS?

#digitalhealth #smartglass #AR #googleglass
The Terminator (1984) Predator (1987)

I like addressing the needs of the elderly and how technology might assist them. After one of my talks a retired gentleman asked whether doctors would literally be able to look through patients in the future. He looked quite worried about the possibility. He thought it might be intimidating for his physician to look into him, "naked" in a new way. Of course, that was not the literal case. I had given examples of how augmented reality works, and I needed to reassure him that it wasn't going to happen soon. It was actually happening already.

Augmented reality allows us to see the world augmented by computer–generated overlays such as sound or video. It merges the real with the digital world into one view. The device can be a mask, a pair of glasses, or even contact lenses.

This field is still very new and under construction. Within three to five years, perhaps, devices will accommodate the user's creativity and come up with practical uses that they can easily customize to their specific needs. Finding a balance between seeing reality and receiving additional digital inputs is tricky. Companies have tried, and many have failed.

Google Glass shows users a screen in the upper right–hand corner of the visual field. You can access calendars, Google searches, and websites, or take still images and videos either with voice control or by swiping your finger on the side of the frame. Dr. Rafael Grossmann was the first surgeon to stream his operation live through Google Glass online. Before only two or three medical students could peek over his shoulder to see what he was doing. Now hundreds of students can watch the operation on a big screen. Glass is not only transforming education but also the doctor–patient visit. The physician can keep eye contact with the patient while inputting or accessing information.

Philips has a similar device that lets surgeons see the patient's vital signs during surgery. This gives them hands–free, voice–controlled access to critical data when needed.

Race Yourself is an augmented reality app for Glass that lets users race against a virtual projection of themselves or someone else such as a friend or celebrity. In game mode they can run from zombies or giants. This could be a great motivation for running. Another app from Britain helps

Parkinson's patients improve their independence by reminding them about medications and contacting relatives in an emergency.

Emergency departments have tested augmented reality for consulting by video with patients who require a dermatologist. Children's Memorial Hermann Hospital in Houston used it to allow children staying at the hospital to remotely "visit" the Houston Zoo.

Google Glass's development was suspended in January 2015. A former Apple designer is rumored to be working on a replacement. Google's focus has shifted from the individual consumer to the industrial user. Glass is not the only device that uses augmented reality. A German hospital in Bremen uses an iPad sealed in sterile bags during operations. The application lets surgeons look into the arteries of an organ as the app merges the picture taken through the camera with the patient's radiology images.

Atheer Labs designed a 3D gesture–controlled augmented reality platform. When I wore these glasses I could open apps and control them with hand gestures I made in front of the glasses. Surgeons could access information from medication allergies to CT scans during an operation without using devices in their hands.

The EyeSeeMed system does not even require wearing eye–tracking glasses. It can detect where the eyes are focused through the use of cameras. Looking at a specific button on the screen for seconds leads to a click to select that option. Tilting the head left and right navigates through radiological images.

Google patented a digital contact lens that can act as a smaller and smarter Google Glass. Imagine controlling what to receive either by voice or perhaps with your thoughts in the future when brain tracking has become common. This technology is not only for physicians. A Canadian inventor has made a bionic lens that can be implanted in a way similar to cataract surgery. The procedure takes 10 minutes, and the lens is designed not to degrade over time. The reason people might want it is that it enhances eyesight to a level three times better than 20/20. Soon we could all have perfect eyesight. Clinical trials will end in 2017.

These kinds of augmented reality devices could let physicians peer into their patients when radiology images are available. It doesn't mean that they will literally see through them, but instead of checking radiology images on a light box they could see them in the context of the patient's anatomy.

Magic Leap is a brave and strange concept, merely an idea backed by a half billion dollars from Google and a team of experts that want to revolutionize the way we use computers. They are developing head–mounted displays that superimpose 3D computer–generated imagery over the real–world scene. The device shines a digital light field onto the user's retina. Open your hands, and a 3D object moves in your hands just like it does on a video. It's hard to imagine that, but the concept videos they have released show the idea's promise.

Microsoft brought out Hololens in 2014 to much fanfare. HoloLens is also a smart glass that projects digital images and data onto the world the user sees. Architecture software that models 3D objects, 3D printer applications, and teaching anatomy are potential uses.

Skype will probably get implemented into HoloLens therefore we could talk to each other in person even though the other person is a continent away. This combination would understand human speech perfectly and follows the user's eye movements. HoloLens can move the cursor to where the user is looking. Microsoft expects it to change everything from work to gaming, even space travel given their collaboration with NASA.

Microsoft had been developing its device for five years before it even announcing its existence. Google, on the other hand, may have erred in coming out with Glass too soon. We will see what future years will bring. I can only be excited about these directions.

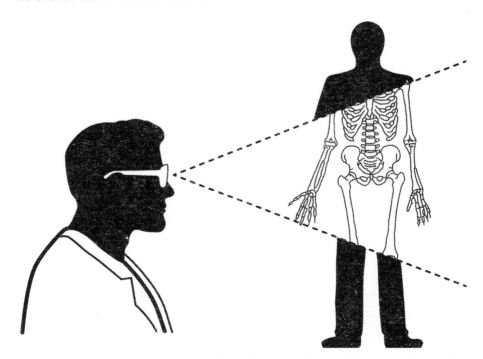

IS PRINTING OUT MEDICAL EQUIPMENT CHEAPER THAN MANUFACTURING?

#digitalhealth #3dprinting | Print The Legend (2014)

After giving a talk at Medicine X, an event organized by Stanford University, a group of young entrepreneurs who were also university students approached me. They wanted to know how they could become medical futurists; which trends I found most exciting; and what I thought about the economic consequences of my views. They were amazed at the potential of 3D printing. Given their own startup, they wanted to know whether printing out medical equipment would be cheaper than manufacturing it with traditional methods. They didn't realize they had answered their own question merely by asking it.

The advantages of medical 3D printing would make a long list. In Dubai I met with Scott Summit, Design Director of 3D Systems. He gave me an unforgettable tour of the various 3D printing solutions they were working on. He told about the daughter of one of the investors who broke her arm. They decided to scan her arm, create a model of the personalized cast she could wear, and printed it out in metal.

Later, when Scott had a wrist problem he took the same approach and quickly scanned his arm with a hand–held object scanner and printed out his own cast. The cost was about $50. But instead of spending hours at the ER or doctor's office, cutting down the traditional cast, checking the arm and getting a new cast; a 3D printed cast could get ready in 2 minutes. His personalized cast can be opened up and closed in seconds. He and the girl were the first patients in history to have a shower with the cast on their broken arms.

A Spanish company, Exovite, is working on making such casts available. They scan the patient's arm, print out a personalized cast in 30 seconds and attach an electrical muscle stimulation device of their own design. A rehabilitation application they developed lets patients control the device, get reminders to do exercises, or seek medical advice from the rehabilitation clinic they are working with.

3D printing works by additive manufacturing. This means that a digital model is created of the object we want to print out, and the machine adds each layer one at a time. Printers can use more than a hundred types of material as "ink". A new method introduced in 2015 prints objects much faster, but the additive manufacturing is still the gold standard.

With advances of 3D printing, dental laboratories and hearing aid manufacturers have started using 3D printers. The end product can be perfectly customized, and the cost is less than manufacturing by traditional means. 3D–produced dental implants fit perfectly the first time because they are manufactured for the mouth of the patient.

Aluminium molds have been traditionally used to make medical prototypes. Using 3D printed molds reduces costs and the time needed to make the final product. It produces prototypes using production–quality materials in 95% less time and 70% less cost than traditional aluminum molds.

A German manufacturer of breast prostheses started using a 3D printer to produce its molds. This resulted in a 50% reduction in costs. Given that they need tools for the different types in 100 different sizes, 3D printing significantly facilitates making them. Before, a wooden template was used to create a prototype. Then they mirrored that in a manual process that took 14 days and resulted in the aluminium mold in which they poured the silicone. Today, they can create any number of digital models and print them out on demand.

Another factor for reducing costs would be making the digital models available to the public. For example, a US research team created a digital library of open source designs for a particular medical device, a syringe pump. Each design is customizable according to needs and can be printed out on demand. Professional syringe pumps used for precise amounts of drug delivery cost hundreds to thousands of dollars. This one can cost $50 per syringe. That is how cost can be reduced and personalization can be added with one new technology.

The FDA is obviously interested in correctly regulating the industry to ensure that 3D printed devices are safe and effective. In 2014 the FDA hosted a public workshop to discuss these issues and provide regulatory standards for 3D–printed devices. As of 2015 the FDA has so far approved 85 medical devices made by 3D printers. These include spinal cages, dental restorative devices, cranial implants, and hearing aids with 3D–printed components.

If you ask people working in the medical device industry, 3D printing will not be new because for them it has been around for decades. Companies realized that creating prototypes is cheaper with 3D printers and therefore gradually started embracing their use. In underdeveloped regions, where even traditional manufacturing is difficult and expensive, groups such as iLab//Haiti have taken to 3D printing umbilical cord clamps for local hospitals in Haiti.

This is what we will see more frequently. Wealthy companies turn to 3D printing because of its potential for total customization. Companies in poorer regions turn to it because it makes prototypes inexpensively. The online community will produce more digital models when 3D printers become common in the home. With a 3D printed prototype, crowdfunding the necessary financial backing will be easier for startups around the world.

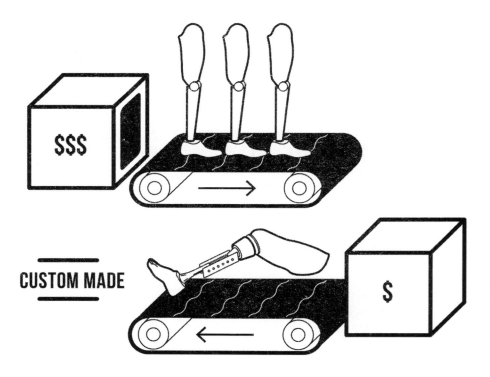

WILL WE EVER TREAT INDIVIDUALS BASED ON THEIR OWN DNA?

#genomics #personalizedmedicine #pm101 | Gattaca (1997)

As a member of the Society of Personalized Medicine I speak every year at general meetings. Researchers in genetics, biotechnology, and bioinformatics attend these events. Physicians also come to hear the latest developments. They are often the most skeptical given that they have to deal with applying the studies to real people. Keeping up with streams of new information is a struggle, and all clinicians have to face it. They can rely on suggestions and policies of organizations that gather and assimilate new clinical information.

One such clinician asked me, in a snarky tone, about using genetic information when making medical decisions every day. As the cost of genome sequencing rapidly diminishes, we will soon all own the data of our personal DNA. Knowledge about the associations between DNA and medical consequences is growing fast. But the intersection between obtaining data and making decisions based on that is still a dark jungle.

The Personalized Medicine Coalition (PMC) has been facilitating this since 2004. I had a chat with Dr. Edward Abrahams, President of PMC. He shared the findings of the 4th edition of the report they published. There are now more than a hundred drugs whose labels include pharmacogenomic information. This means that studies have found associations between genetic aspects and sensitivity to that particular drug.

For example, physicians need to check for two DNA variations before prescribing a drug to prevent venous blood clotting. One variation makes the patient more sensitive to a standard dose; the other metabolizes the drug faster than normal. If someone with either of these DNA variations received the standard dose that works for the general population, they would have side effects that might require hospitalization.

According to the PMC database we know of more than 50 million DNA variations, thousands of which are associated with specific drugs and diseases. In cancer, certain tumors are driven by genetic mutations that could be targets for specific drugs. Melanoma, thyroid, and colon cancers are among the most responsive tumors. Drugs are ineffective for about 40% of patients with asthma, depression, and diabetes. It has nothing to do with the quality of the drug or the physician's treatment plan, but the fact that we are all genetically unique. This shouldn't be surprising given that we have 3 billion base pairs in our DNA.

Personalized medicine means getting only the treatments that are customized to our genetic and metabolic backgrounds. To initiate this we need to obtain our personal DNA data. Thousands of people already have it either because they paid enormous amounts of money for what is now a $2,500 prospect, or because they were subjects in a study. Over a million people who purchased direct–to–consumer genetic tests also own a portion of their DNA. To make DNA sequencing widely available, costs must come down to that of standard blood markers.

Storage is another problem, and a bigger one that one would think. DNA sequencing generates terabytes of information per person. Do this for billions of individuals, and who knows how many associations and studies will need to be stored and analyzed. That is a true big data challenge. Thinking linearly we might think in terms of larger hard drives. But Google has started working on a genomics division that will store one person's genome in the cloud for $25 a year.

In 2014 the National Cancer Institute said it would pay $19 million to move copies of the 2.6 petabyte Cancer Genome Atlas from several thousand cancer patients into the cloud. It would allow researchers to use this huge data trove to run virtual experiments whenever they wanted to test a genetic association. Imagine a potential scenario: a cancer patient gets a diagnosis. Their genome and their tumor's genome are inexpensively sequenced right away. The data sets are then compared to millions of others belonging to similar patients with similar tumors whose outcomes are already known. That would be a gold mine of information pertinent to patient care.

A company called DeCode Genetics based in Iceland has collected the sequences of more than 10,000 island residents who are closely related. From these, they could extrapolate the DNA makeup of the other 320,000 inhabitants on the island. This way the company discovered that thousands of people carry a genetic mutation that increases the risk for breast and ovarian cancer. They have been debating with health authorities whether to notify them or not. Let's stop here for a second. A company based on large genetic datasets can tell people what conditions they may face soon or what conditions they should specifically try to prevent. What is personalized healthcare if not this?

Of course, privacy is a huge issue and many people resist sequencing for this reason. They don't want to share their DNA information with anyone.

It's a hard decision. If I had to disclose my DNA in order to receive useful alerts about my future health, I'm in. But again, this must be a personal decision.

The final concern is interpretation. This might be the trickiest part. How does one draw medical conclusions from the massive databases and an individual's genetic makeup and lifestyle? Introducing genomic medicine in the current medical school curriculum might help. But decisions about every patient must be personalized just as their genetic background is.

The PMC report spoke of a physician who tells his patients that genetic knowledge is power. It isn't about good news or bad news. It is about understanding the underlying cause of disease and using it to tailor a plan of prevention. This is what genomic information can provide us with. Every treatment can be personalized at the time a treatment decision is made. Shaping such personalized treatments has been happening in healthcare for more than a decade, but not for everyone and not everywhere. The US Precision Medicine Initiative encourages customizing care through research, and technology to make that treatment more targeted.

Getting a specific drug in a dosage tailored to my biological details is amazing. But if we had learned at the time of the completion of the Human Genome Project that there were only going to be around a hundred examples in practice by 2015, we might have been disappointed. Perhaps expectations were too high. There still is a way to go until my DNA will contribute as much to my care as a blood test or my lifestyle.

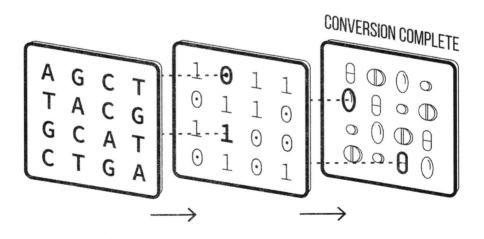

CONVERSION COMPLETE

FOR HOW LONG WILL WE TEST DRUGS ON ACTUAL PEOPLE?

#digitalhealth #clinicaltrial | S1m0ne (2002)

I honestly hate sitting on panel discussions. I like offering solutions to problems, and such discussions rarely provide a chance for that. Still, I accept invitations and sit on these panels with the thought that you never know when you'll get a challenging question. At an event organized by the pharmaceutical industry, I sat with representatives from major pharma companies. I had given a talk about how disruptive innovations would transform the pharma industry entirely. To my surprise there were patients in the audience.

One patient directed his question about human testing to another member of the panel. I was glad, because I covered the issue in my talk and wanted to hear what pharma representatives had to say about it. Current pharma models involve a lengthy and expensive process of clinical trials whose purpose is to assess the safety and efficacy of potential new drugs.

New drugs are approved through human clinical trials. These are rigorous, starting in animal trials and gradually moving to patients. It typically costs billions of dollars and takes many years to complete, sometimes more than a decade. Patients in trials are exposed to side effects that cannot be predicted or expected. If the trial is successful, it may or may not receive FDA approval.

Online services have helped clinical trials. TrialReach tries to bridge the gap between patients and researchers who are developing new drugs. If more patients have a chance to participate in trials, they might become more engaged with potential treatments or even be able to access new treatments before they become FDA approved and freely available. TrialX similarly matches clinical trials to patients according to their gender, age, location, and medical condition. The number of such services is growing to accommodate an increasing demand from patients.

In the late 19th century patients had no protection. Anyone could sell snake oil containing who–knows–what. In 1906, the FDA was born and required every tonic, nostrum, and product to be tested and proven both safe and efficient. While an extremely important element of healthcare today, it puts immense economic pressure to bear on bringing new treatments to market.

If a pharmaceutical company jumps through all the hoops and wins approval, they can sell their new product for a limited time under patent protection. If it does not win approval, all their investment goes down the drain. Some patient activists are arguing that the process should be changed. For example, Perry Cohen, a Parkinson's disease patient, has argued for years that the FDA has been using the wrong criteria. As he sees it the question is for whose benefit trials are being done, and who gets to say what that benefit means.

Obviously, we a need a faster and less expensive method that is also safe. What if it's time to use disruptive innovations to change how clinical trials are performed? We need to mimic human physiology digitally for this which is hard. Fortunately, we are not imitating the end product, and so while mimicking human physiology is extremely difficult it is not totally impossible. A comprehensive system would make it possible to model conditions, symptoms, and even drug effects. To achieve this, every tiny detail of the human body needs to be included in the simulation– from the way we react to temperature changes to the circadian rhythms that influence the action of hormones.

HumMod is one of the most advanced simulations. It provides a top–down model of human physiology from whole organs to individual molecules. It features more than 1,500 equations and 6,500 variables such as body fluids, circulation, electrolytes, hormones, metabolism, and skin temperature. Hum-Mod aims to simulate how human physiology works, and claims to be the most sophisticated mathematical model of human physiology ever created.

HumMod has been in development for decades and it is still far from completion. By far, I mean perhaps decades still. There are those who argue that human physiology cannot be digitally imitated. Maybe supplementary technologies are needed such as organ microchips. For example, organs–on–chips are engineered to mimic how the lung or the heart works at the cellular level. They are translucent, and so can provide a window into the inner workings of a particular organ.

The Wyss Institute plans to build ten different organs–on–chips and connect them together. Doing this may mimic whole–body physiology better, and thus better assess responses to new drug candidates.

Imagine if we could test thousands of new potential drugs on billions of virtual patient models in minutes? What would it take to achieve such a capability? At the very least, the virtual patients must almost perfectly mimic the physiology of the target patients, with all of the variation that actual patients show. The model should encompass circulatory, neural, endocrine, and metabolic systems, and each of these must demonstrate valid mechanism–based responses to physiological and pharmacological stimuli. Probably cognitive computers would be needed to deal with the gargantuan amount of resulting data.

All possible variations combining thousands of elements could reveal really complicated patterns. Clinical trials would never be the same.

After the members of the panel had tried to break the question of human testing into smaller pieces, I jumped in and said I hoped that technology will soon allow us to test drugs not on patients but in silica. You might assume that developing the supercomputers for this or simulating the wonderfully complex human body on a chip are the biggest challenges to bring this about. But I think the biggest obstacle will be the resistance of pharma companies and authorities that don't like to change a very old process.

The increasing number of empowered patients who want to be there when their treatments are designed and decided upon might be able to facilitate to change this. Let's hope I'm not right about big pharma's resistance, and that they will want to be among the first companies to turn their attention toward disrupting clinical trials. If the incentives become clear, and there are investment opportunities then the change will happen faster than we think. If not, empowered patients may decide to start their own clinical trials.

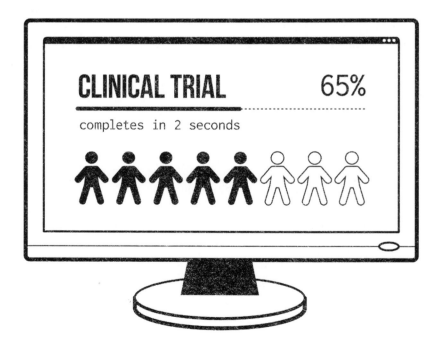

WHAT WILL THE HOSPITAL OF THE FUTURE LOOK LIKE?

#digitalhealth #hospital #HIMSS | The Fifth Element (1997)

It's not so hard to find me online, therefore I get a lot of messages on several social media channels. I once received a very polite e–mail from a student who was studying modern architecture. He was working on his thesis and his topic was the hospital of the future. He had found plenty of articles articulating my views about this. He invited me to coffee and asked me to forget any rules I knew. He wanted to me design a hospital that would be completely digital, tech oriented, and futuristic.

I said it wasn't that simple. Many institutions had already tried to de-sign such a hospital. Moreover, I wasn't totally sure that in the future we'll need hospitals like the ones we have now. I couldn't tell which surprised him more. Healthcare is built around hospitals mainly because medical expertise and equipment have only been accessible there. But that's not the case anymore.

I consulted John Sharp, Senior Manager at the Healthcare Informa-tion and Management Systems Society (HIMSS), because he has been a spokesman for digital health for years. He agreed with these surprising trends. Some US hospitals are new, elegant facilities that look more like hotels than traditional hospitals. Others, particularly small community hospitals, are clos-ing their doors from lack of demand. The slack demand for inpatient beds will shift care to outpatient facilities and homes. Because of this the hospital of the future will probably be intensive care units and post–surgery recovery facilities.

These facilities will be enhanced with high tech devices and broad data availability projected on large screens and mobile devices. Rooms will accommodate families and technology seamlessly. For instance, hospital room TVs will be flat screens for entertainment and patient education. But they will also let the care team call up images and data to explain the patient's case to both the family and patient. Mobile devices, like tablets, will be in the hands of providers as well as patients so that they can record their pain, for example, other symptoms, and contact the nursing station. Some pilot projects like this already exist.

More care will shift to the home setting as technology becomes avail-able to manage it there. Different types of monitors are already available, and hospitals are experimenting with using these to prevent readmissions of chronically ill and high risk patients such as those with congestive heart failure. As we move toward the Internet of Things, more of these monitoring devices will become embedded in homes and be the norm rather than the exception. There will still be a need for nurse practitioners and nurse's aides, but even they will become a technical resource for patients—something like a "Geek Squad" for home health technology.

This entails some obvious risks. Sharp heard of one patient who was sent home with chemotherapy programmed into his pump. But the pump was not programmed correctly, and a serious mishap occurred. Examples like this demonstrate why standards for home health technology will need to be tightened, and why hands—on assistance in the home will need to be assessed on a case—by—case basis.

Designing a hospital of the future doesn't start with futuristic technologies. The best examples of hospitals that exploit digital solutions are those that are designed in cooperation with patients. If patients are being asked to take more initiative in their care via technology like mobile devices, then they should be involved in designing the user interface, and testing the apps that go with it. One can also recruit patient navigators to assist those with chronic conditions in navigating the healthcare system, and also pilot through electronic data intended for patient education.

The hospital of the future might benefit from some current trends: augmented reality glasses, walls that project a virtual reality so that patients literally feel as if they are at home, 3D printers and more that can render care less expensively and more efficiently. Portable radiology devices will communicate wirelessly with other devices. Minimal waiting times brought about by cognitive computers that organize logistics will result in better quality of life. It will direct people when and where to go by analyzing their records, and automatically responding to doctors' notes and prescriptions. Robots will move freely about, engaging either in telemedical services or disinfecting rooms in seconds.

Some of these examples are already in practice. Carolinas Health-Care System has a smartphone app through which patients can access medical care information on demand. The Duke Institute for Health Innovation sponsored a competition to address three areas: medical complications, primary care, and population health and analytics. The Ochsner Health System designed the O bar, similar to Apple's genius bar in their retail stores. It demonstrates tablets, flat screen TVs, and wearable devices all in an effort to improve patient education. The first wholly digital, paperless hospital is set to open in the United Arab Emirates in 2015. Consultants from the prestigious Cleveland Clinic helped them design it.

The largest segment of healthcare is actually self–care, which takes place outside of the medical system. Patients need to manage their health and disease not only in the hospital and during the doctor visits, but also at home. Still, when people talk about the future of hospitals, they imagine space–age technologies and gigantic machines. But what if the majority of care could be provided in our homes? What if wearable devices could measure what needs to be measured in the comfort of our bathroom or bedroom? What if smart clothes and brain activity trackers could change the way in which we telecommute and work from home?

The bathroom could feature a smart scale that measures your weight, percentage of body fat, lean muscle mass, bone density, BMI, and degree of hydration, and then recognizes who you are and sends the data to your smartphone. Your bathroom mirror could be a digital one that assesses your stress level, pulse, and emotional mood when you look into it. It could offer you news clips relevant to what it finds. Your smart toothbrush could tell whether you were sufficiently hydrated, and reward you for spending enough time brushing. The toilet might contain a microchip that performs urine analysis. Before you step into the shower your smart home will bring the temperature up to the level you prefer via a simple device like the Nest thermostat.

The bedroom could feature smart sleep monitors that wake you up at the most auspicious time so that you feel rested and energized for the day ahead. In the morning the monitors would report your sleep quality. When you retire to bed, your smart sleep monitor will let your Nest thermostat know that it should lower the temperature because sleep is most sound and restful when the bedroom is cool. Sleep monitors might activate specific music and lighting programs to gently wake you up. Pulse, pulse variability, breathing, and oxygen saturation could also be measured to reduce the incidence of sleep apnea and snoring.

Turning to the kitchen, one might find smart forks and spoons that either prompt us to eat slowly, or let individuals with Parkinson's disease counteract the disruptive effects of their tremor so that they can feed themselves again. Various scanners could measure ingredients, allergens, and potential toxins in our food, and let smartphone applications help control our diet. 3D food printers loaded with fresh ingredients might create pizzas, cookies, or any kind of products just like the Foodini currently does.

The hospital of the future will represent care of the future. Whether it takes place at home, or in a place we still call the hospital, what matters is that patients take an active part in accessing the information they need. Today's patients need access to the hospital. Tomorrow, hospitals will be designed around patients.

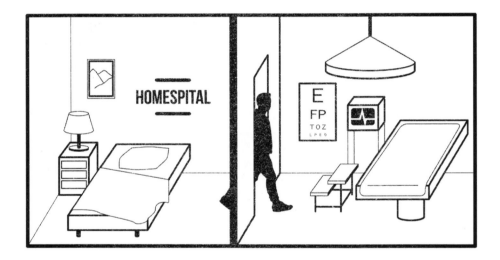

WILL VIRTUAL REALITY TAKE OVER OUR LIVES?

#virtualreality #cardboard #vr | Surrogates (2009)

Sometimes I alarm people with the possibilities I describe. The examples I talk about make them uncomfortable. People don't like change, and what I show them is a world full of changes. No matter how hard I try to present workable and optimistic solutions, they are still plain scared. Talking to people who are not that tech savvy is an even bigger challenge. For example, I agreed to speak to hundreds of pensioners in Budapest in 2014. Organizers said they were open to everything, and that they wanted my talk to focus on the importance of health management. I gave only mild examples, but still some in the audience became worried.

A man in his 70s raised his hand to ask a question. He rambled on for a long time about how he struggles with technology. Finally, he asked if virtual reality was going to take over our lives. He seemed really worried about the possibility. I told him it would not. But we will all have to decide for ourselves.

My first experience with virtual reality was Google Cardboard. This is a fold–out cardboard with two lenses. By inserting your smartphone with a specific application running on it, you can feel as if you are in a virtual world. The app has split images, one for each eye, which is how your brain turns it into a virtual reality. Cardboard was introduced at a tech conference in 2014, and costs around $20. I downloaded an app that lets me roam around the castle of Versailles. The quality wasn't perfect but it did feel like I was there. I showed it to my 7 year–old niece who said she'd like to have the real experience after seeing Versailles like that.

There are apps designed to experience Jurassic Parks, huge swings, cosmic distances flying around planets and even real–life movies in 3D. Once you see how Cardboard creates a virtual reality, you will be tempted to access more advanced applications. One of the earliest examples of a successfully crowdfunded project, Oculus Rift, was later acquired by Facebook. It will let you share not only your photos and status updates, but also whatever environment you are in. You put on the Oculus Rift, save the 360 degree images around you, and let your friends see exactly what you see when you look around. It will be available in 2016.

MetaVR software creates PC–based virtual worlds. They sell both the hardware and software required for users to create their own virtual worlds.

Project Morpheus from Sony is a headset, to be released in 2016, that will focus on gaming and connect a Playstation controller to the headset. Expect to see people riding the subway putting on their headsets and playing while they commute to work. Currently we may be diving into our smartphone screens, but soon we will literally be diving into deep water with virtual reality headsets.

In Dubai at a digital health conference I tried on a head display developed by Samsung. It was designed to train anesthesiologists. I literally felt like I was in the operating room, with the staff talking about the patient's case. I could see them in high definition. A few years ago I had studied from old books with small print. Now I could train as long as I wanted in the comfort of my home.

Physicians learn to do procedures by repetition. In March 2015, surgeons explored the potential of virtual reality by capturing interventional procedures with a special 360 degree camera. The recordings were then transformed into a format that could be used with virtual reality headsets. Having a chance to see an experienced professional do a procedure over and over by standing next to him or her virtually can be useful for students. The "see one, do one, teach one" method of conventional medical training is outdated. We need to give students the chance to get better at a procedure without the equipment and time limitations of medical education. We cannot ask patients to be around so students can gather experience all the time. But students can use virtual reality to do the same. I can watch how to take a blood sample a hundred times before I do one for real. That is a benefit for everyone.

A company called Next Galaxy is working on a digital environment that lets health professionals train in resuscitation. They think virtual reality represents the highest form of learning because the user is immersed in the task and actually doing it, rather than watching someone else doing it on a video.

It could also provide a new form of engagement in rehabilitation. GestureTek Health's virtual reality therapies aim to make the process of stretching physical and cognitive capabilities fun. They are working with cerebral palsy, stroke, traumatic injuries, autism, and similar conditions.

People who fear public speaking can train with virtual reality headsets that place them in front of thousands of people. Patients struggling with addiction could see what the world would look like if they could beat their addiction. While attending a conference in California I heard about a woman who had a serious fear of spiders. She vacuumed her bed for an hour each night. Psychologists worked with her by creating a virtual world in which she was introduced to tiny spiders and then gradually larger and larger ones. I saw a photo of her with a giant tarantula spider sitting on her arm one year after therapy started.

The future of the medical curriculum will definitely include virtual reality. Students will be trained to respond efficiently during stressful, emergency situations, to which they will be exposed throughout their medical school years. Wearable sensors might give them immediate feedback as to how they perform.

Physicians could virtually enter inside their patient based on radiology images. This way they could discover various options before cutting the patient in the operating room. We could train people for emergency and disaster situations without risking real lives. If one has no available cadaver on which to practice surgery, then virtual reality can help.

Patients could sample the hospital experience before arrival. They could see how a given procedure takes place, how much time it takes, what's going to happen to them. Head displays could relieve stress by letting people experience the real world through virtual reality.

Those who have not tried virtual reality cannot imagine how hard it is going to be to persuade people to keep living their lives without such devices. The brain is easily tricked. Virtual reality might just become the new drug of the future. A 2014 study actually compared addiction to virtual reality technology to addiction to hard drugs. When will we be tempted to give up reality for the virtual kind?

On the positive side, video gamers might soon become the athletes of the future. Devices exist that let users experience virtual reality by wearing a headset attached to a half sphere in which they safely walk or run. This area is called exergaming. In this way they can only advance in the game if they exercise in real life. Football games, first–person shooters, and even strategy games could motivate users to exercise more than ever before. Current cinema and television films depict hardcore gamers as lazy people who sit in front of their computer, eat doughnuts, and are obese. Given that virtual reality is becoming more real and requires greater activity on the part of the user, obesity might have a brand new enemy.

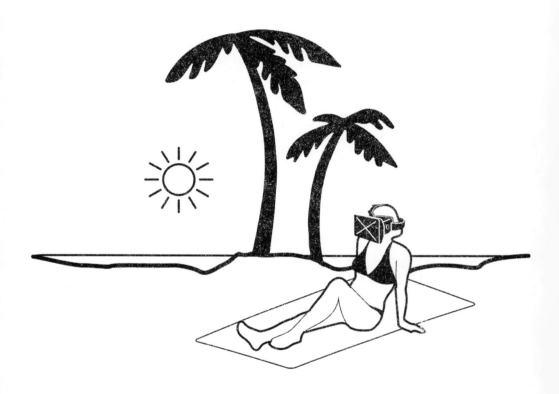

WILL THERE BE OPERATING ROOMS MANNED ONLY WITH ROBOTS?

#surgicalrobots #intuitivesurgical | Prometheus (2012)

The Kairos Society works with young entrepreneurs to develop ideas that can affect a lot of people. Given that one never knows who might be the next brilliant innovator in medicine, I gladly accepted the invitation of the Kairos Society's local branch to speak about the use of robots in healthcare. I love giving presentations on narrow topics because it gives me an opportunity to learn new things. I immersed myself in the world of medical and surgical robots, and at the conference there was a lively discussion about their advantages and potential threats. A young attendee asked whether there would ever be operating rooms staffed only by robots. My answer was simple given that such operating rooms already exist, although there are not many of them.

The term robot in our vernacular comes from Czech playwright Karel Capek's 1920 play, R.U.R, or Rossum's Universal Robots (Rosumovi Univerzální Roboti). The word robot means "worker". In the 1970s, NASA needed to design robots that could do surgery and yet be controlled remotely. The first such surgical robot made its appearance during a laparoscopic surgery in 1987. Since then, only one company has made a commercially available and widely popular surgical robot. It's called Intuitive Medical and its robot goes under the name da Vinci. One robot costs over $1 million, but the economic aspect of its business model pertains to service and providing additional tools. Such robots still require human supervision.

Surgeons sit behind a control panel. They can move the robot's arms within a 3–dimensional virtual reality space. Cameras mounted on the articulated arms let the doctors make the tiniest movement with confidence using joystick controls. A number of medical schools have started teaching the skills required for operating via surgical robot. Compared to traditional surgical skills, these resemble those of video gamers. Studies suggest that surgeons who have a history of having played video games perform tasks via the surgical robots with a smaller error percentage than others.

The Raven Surgical Robotic System is similar. NASA has included it in its trials since 2009. Its overall mass is only 22 kg, much lower than that of da Vinci. In 2015 Google announced a collaboration with Johnson & Johnson. They plan to design robots assisting surgeons. Google stated it planned to use its machine–vision and image–analysis softwares to help make the robot. Nobody knows how fast they can break into this market, but there are no doubts they will.

I had the opportunity to use a Nintendo Wii console that had been reengineered to teach the skills that surgeons use while performing laparoscopic operations. I learned by playing. When I sat in front of the da Vinci control panel as a video gamer I didn't need instruction as to how to move the robot's arms. Give me a joystick and I will deal with it. Of course doing surgery involves professional training, but the skills are different than before. Using a scalpel and controlling a robot require different trainings. I heard surgeons talking about cases during which the surgical robot stopped working and the surgeon had to resume traditional methods. It can be struggle for those who were trained merely for controlling robots.

Surgical robots are not intended to substitute for either surgeons or traditional methods. They are meant to assist. Not every procedure is amenable to robots and those that are controlled by attending surgeons. For obvious reasons a procedure slated to be performed entirely by a robot must go through a great deal of quality control.

VascuLogic has developed a robot to make blood collection safer and more efficient. It takes the blood sample autonomously while the patient sits comfortably. Infrared and ultrasound imaging guides the needle into a vein. The company claims that its robotic venipuncture is a less painful and safer method than a human phlebotomist. A 2015 video demonstrates the machine in action. Before it is allowed in general use it will have to go through many steps of a clinical trial.

More than half a million surgical robots exist worldwide. Because they lack the possibility of human error, they are considered safer than traditional methods even though they cost more than traditional equipment. In 2004, there were 13.3 injuries or deaths per 100,000 procedures caused by a machine. This rose to 50 in 2012. In recent years hundreds of cases of robotic injuries have been reported to the FDA. And the cost–quality ratio is still under investigation. It could be safer but it costs much more than procedures before. These are the issues we have to take into consideration.

Robots will need to get better at performing specific tasks given that there are tens of thousands of potential procedures that a robot could do or assist with. Their size will shrink either because of better materials or manufacturing cheap parts with 3D printers. Maintenance costs will diminish–currently a large factor in robot profitability.

Robotic safety should be the number one issue. A surgical robot was controlled remotely from a distance for the first time in 2001. A surgeon in New York operated remotely on a patient in Strasbourg, France, a distance of 6,000 kilometers. The communication between controller and robot took place through public Internet networks.

This unfortunately opens up possibilities for hackers. In 2015, researchers at the University of Washington showed that a malicious attacker could disrupt a telerobot during surgery. Hackers could take over control from a distance. The robot in question has not been approved by the FDA. But still it raises issues that we will have to deal with in order to ensure patient safety.

With respect to safety issues there are plans for tethered robots, tiny machines whose parts can be swallowed and assembled in the stomach where they then remotely perform minor operations. What happens if such a robot is hacked or hijacked remains unknown.

Companies are focusing on improving features in coming generations of robots. If telerobots can operate efficiently and safely without immediate human presence, then perhaps patients could be in a room populated with only robots while those are still controlled by surgeons from a different location. This way surgical care could be provided to people living in areas with doctor shortages; and infections during operations could be significantly reduced. The ultimate goal is including touch feedback. Surgeons could feel the patient's skin through the controllers just like they do in traditional operations today.

In the 19th century surgeons sat in large lecture halls and watched operations live to learn new surgical methods. Surgery was more like do–it–yourself handiwork that used very basic tools. Today, surgery is a set of laser–precise movements and quick decisions. In many types of operations the patient goes to the hospital in the morning, gets operated on, and leaves on the same day. Making even complicated surgeries as painless and comfortable as possible, and promoting fast recovery is a top goal of providers. When this is available to patients worldwide, we will have enough time to worry about robots taking over operating rooms.

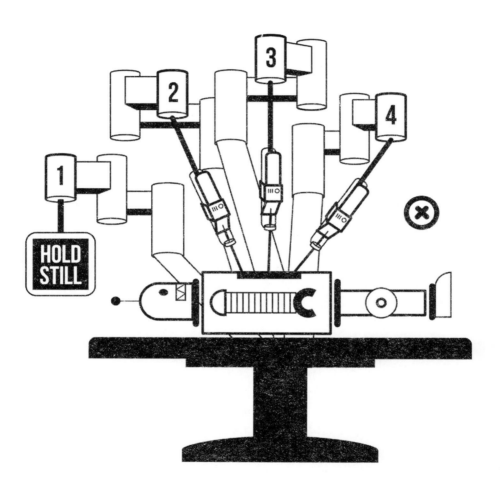

CAN AN ALGORITHM DIAGNOSE BETTER THAN A DOCTOR?

#digitalhealth #ibmwatson I Her (2013) Ex Machina (2015)

I'm not an engineer, unfortunately. Giving talks to engineers is a challenge because I almost never focus on the things they are the most interested in. Even as a geek, I don't enjoy diving into the technical details of a new solution. I'm interested in its application in practice and in further developing it. Once when I spoke to engineering students at a university, the discussion afterward got a bit heated. They didn't seem to care about basic ethical issues, or the advantages of disruptive technologies.

They wanted to know the hard stuff. Most of their questions focused on physicians being replaced by robots. I emphasized the importance of empathy and the personal relationship between physician and patient based on trust, but at one point they got me. They asked whether algorithms could theoretically be better at making a diagnosis than doctors.

I was in trouble. With my doctor's cap on, I must defend the art of medicine. But as a medical futurist I need to tell my honest views. Making a diagnosis is an art. We are not engineering products, and therefore measuring a few parameters and changing a few things will not diagnose and cure any disease. Instead, physicians are trained to look at the whole human being from head to toe. The way the patient walks, speaks, smells, or thinks are all important to the final diagnosis. That is one part of the equation.

The other part is learning and gathering whatever information is relevant to the patient's case. Being a physician entails a commitment towards life–long learning. They dive into biomedical databases of peer–reviewed papers, and find the information they need. Keeping up-to-date with the latest literature in our field of interest is normal routine in the life of a physician.

The first part is what improves with experience, and technologies might never replace that. Wearable devices and home monitoring services can measure a lot of parameters, but the physician's first impression on meeting a patient is irreplaceable.

The other part is where everybody fails. No doctor in the world can be perfectly up–to–date. No doctor can be certain they have found all the pertinent information their case requires. This is a matter of luck right now, and we should remove this factor of luck from the practice of medicine.

To do so we need help from the world of technology.

In 1996, the IBM supercomputer Deep Blue challenged Garry Kasparov, the reigning world chess champion. Kasparov won, and headlines around the world celebrated the triumph of humanity over the computer. IBM used the experience from the match to improve Deep Blue's algorithms, and asked for a re–match in 1997. Kasparov lost to Deep Blue this time, 2.5 to 3.5. Kasparov argued that if he had had access to the same databases as the computer, he could have won the match.

Based on Kasparov's suggestion a new form of chess match format was introduced in Spain in 1998. Advanced Chess players played against one another by using chess softwares. The human player decides on the move, but the human–software pairing is considered a team. This is a winning combination of human creativity and the powerful computing.

Watson, IBM's new supercomputer, aims to fill this gap. After it beat two highly skilled players in the television quiz show *Jeopardy*, US clinics started testing its application in the practice of medicine. The advantage Watson offers is an ability to comb through patient records, English textbooks, and millions of medical papers in existing databases. Its algorithms arrive at diagnostic suggestions, and assign probable success rates to them. In the end the treating physician makes the decision assisted with pertinent information gleaned by Watson.

Two features of Watson are noteworthy. It employs natural language processing, meaning it can understand written and spoken language. It also uses deep question–and–answer technology. It can enter into conversation and learn more during it. Given that medical practices use different electronic medical records, Watson must be able to understand both structured and unstructured data. Some physicians take notes about a diabetes patient, mentioning "diabetes" or "T1D" in the clinical summary. Understanding natural language means distinguishing between a note that is important and one that is not in a given context.

I was not surprised when the MD Anderson Cancer Center announced it would start using Watson. In oncology, a mountain of studies is published every day. Finding information relevant to a particular patient's case is difficult no matter how much experience the treating physician has. When Watson goes over the patient's case, it comes up with the list of suggestions for treatment and assigns a confidence value between very low and very high. MD Anderson researchers evaluated Watson's success rates and found it to be very efficient. Because physicians rate the suggestions that Watson comes up with, it improves with each case.

In May 2015, a collaboration between Watson, Epic – a software company focusing on electronic health records – and the Mayo Clinic began. Epic has 350 customers that exchange over 80 million medical records annually. The Mayo Clinic has more than 1 million patient visits a year and conducts at least a thousand clinical trials at any time. Using Watson to analyze that huge amount of data or answer the questions of patients seems like a good step forward. One Mayo Clinic oncologist called Watson's potential to provide clinical trial information wherever is needed crucial.

A supercomputer becomes a cognitive computer when it tries to reproduce behavior of the human brain through artificial intelligence. Human physiology is so complex that we can benefit from computers that mimic the way we think and pose questions. Such computers improve by learning just as physicians do–except they improve more quickly.

Can an algorithm diagnose more accurately than a physician? There is no reason to believe it won't be able to, although a few decades will still be needed for that. Would such algorithms replace doctors then? I highly doubt it. Their role will change but they will always be needed. If you ask patients whether they want to be treated by a computer or a person, the majority will choose the person. We are social beings. We need to discuss our health issues not only for the sake of receiving proper treatment, but also because words alone can heal.

There is no algorithm or smartphone app for empathy or understanding. Don't doubt that there will be some that mimic the way we provide empathy, but this is not the direction of current developments. We need algorithms that help physicians find the best options. Cognitive computing can bring all the information into care that we need.

For the first time in history, making a decision about a patient's case will not be based on luck but on pure information and informed decision–making. I honestly don't care if my physician working alone or with an algorithm finds the best solution for my health problem. I care even less whether cognitive computers are used to provide care if my physician can focus on me instead of keyboards and monitors. The practice of medicine remains an art, but its colors can be mixed by an algorithm if the painter is still human.

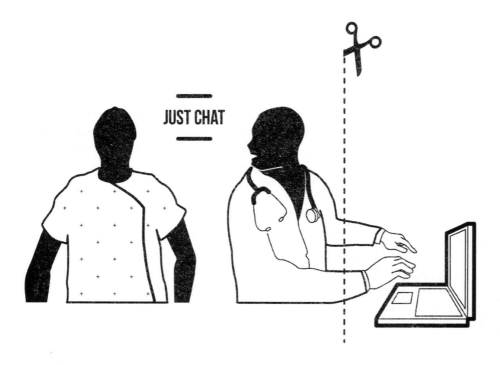

JUST CHAT

CHAPTER 3. AND BEYOND

WILL WE BE ABLE TO TRANSMIT OR READ THOUGHTS?

#digitalhealth #neuroscience | eXistenZ (1999)
Eternal Sunshine of the Spotless Mind (2004)

I constantly look for practical solutions when coming up against a challenge. Discussing futuristic potentials and scenarios is great, but finding a solution that can be put into practice is what matters. I struggle when someone invites me to talk about the distant future. As a science fiction fan I'm happy to imagine how cyborgs, brain implants, and artificial intelligence will transform our lives fully knowing that these speculations won't help people who are living today.

After one of these "And beyond" presentations I have given, an audience member asked whether we will be able to transmit or at least read thoughts. In addition, he said it would be great if he could understand what his wife wants when they have a fight. The audience laughed.

I thought he was referring to an experiment conducted by Dr. Kevin Warwick in which his hand and his wife's were electronically wired together remotely through implanted arrays. The man in the audience was serious although badly misinformed, as reading thoughts is not a new idea. Movies such as *Dune*, *Star Wars*, *X–Men* and even the comedy *What Women Want* depict the consequences and methods of reading thoughts.

Dr. Warwick didn't start experimenting with his wife, but with himself. In 2001 he implanted a chip under his skin and tried to connect his nervous system electronically to computers to move a robotic arm. The signal produced was detailed enough to successfully move it. When he connected the nervous systems of his and his wife's to each other through electrodes, it was supposed to be the first step towards a future form of telepathy. It was the first direct and purely electronic communication between the nervous systems of two persons. When they checked the microchip implants, it seemed nervous tissue didn't reject it. Instead, they saw the tissue grow around the electrode enclosing the sensors. That was Project Cyborg which is still far from telepathy but it showed connecting a nervous system to an electronic one might be possible in the future.

A few things are still missing to be able to read and transmit thoughts electronically. We must be able to perfectly understand how the brain works. We need a device to read electronic signal from the brain without noise.

And there should be a method to transcribe those signals back into conceivable thoughts again. None of this is possible today.

In order to understand structures and creatures, we usually simulate their processes and elements with computers. When a system only consists of a small number of these, it is a matter of time. A worm called C. Elegans that is often the subject of neural studies has 302 neurons. The human brain has about 100 billion neurons that make approximately 100 trillion connections. It means every neuron has about 1,000 connections. It's obvious this is not only a matter of computational power. The complex brain is not simply the summary of how the 100 billion neurons work and communicate. The human brain is more than that.

Ray Kurzweil famously predicted that the computational capacity of an affordable computing device will be approximately equal to the computational capability of the human brain by 2019. It equals 20 quadrillion calculations per second. You don't want to know how big a number that is. If he is right, although many of his predictions have failed already, we would understand how the vast majority of brain functions work biologically. Signs of this have been around for years.

A machine in a lab in Berkeley, California can tell what the subject is looking at by reading off electrical signals of their brain. Its creators suggested in 2008 that in a few decades' time, we would eventually be able to read dreams. Four years later, a computer in a Japanese lab predicted the content of hallucinations at a 60% accuracy using MRI technique. DARPA is working on SyNAPSE, a hardware reconstruction of a human brain that should be ready by 2019.

Understanding how the brain works is not just a question of research. Amazing computers are needed to simulate the vast number of processes. The race for the fastest supercomputer is analogue to the space race in the 1960s. The fastest supercomputer, Tianhe–2, is in China, and it can perform one thousand trillion operations per second. It's still 3–fold away from the brain though. The Department of Energy in the US will spend $200 million to build the fastest one by 2018. Let's assume that with current developments, the discovery of all brain functions and their background is going to be almost complete in a decade.

The next step is the device that reads electric signals of the brain efficiently. When I asked Conor Russomanno, Co–Founder of OpenBCI, about this, he said that reading thoughts is too complex to be described with a single phrase. It's not so black and white. Meaningful and valuable information can be extracted through a non–invasive human–computer interface. Things such as focus and alertness can be derived from a simple EEG system with just a few electrodes. In the context of other data from eye–tracking and location to heart rate and heart rate variability or recorded moods and activities, this data become much more interesting and valuable.

As more invasive forms of brain–computer interfacing continue to develop, the ability to read thoughts will take on a new meaning. We'll be able to look at the brain in much higher resolution and with a lot less noise, at which point the ability to reverse–engineer a specific thought will seem much more realistic. Obviously there are a number of ethical things to consider with this approach. Privacy, security, safety, social stratification, and other issues must be considered as design constraints.

This research direction will clearly be most beneficial to paralyzed individuals. A brain implant could restore the damaged or lost function of the brain to control limbs. If not damaged limbs, then it will control robotic arms. This technology has been demonstrated numerous times, and the media doesn't cover new developments because it's not novelty any longer. Technical difficulties remain with the silicone sensors, although it seems that the organic–electrochemical transistors could make an efficient connection between the surface of the brain and silicon electronics.

If brain implants let paralyzed people walk again or control robotic limbs with their thoughts, it will not mean that we can finally read another person's thoughts. These tasks may be achieved fairly easily, but reading thoughts and dreams is, from a theoretical perspective, far more complicated and remains in the realm of fantasy. Although it would be arrogant to conclude that simulations and cognitive computers will not mimic our human brain. Maybe we will soon digitalize our thoughts. But reality is way behind our imagination on this. I'm not taking a big risk saying that this is not something I should worry about in the coming decade or so. And a lot of patients would benefit from me being wrong.

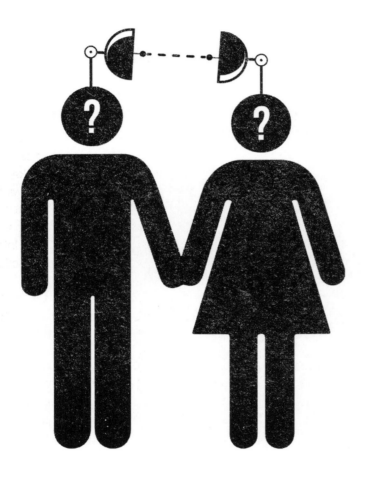

WHAT MAKES SOMEONE A CYBORG?

#cyborg #medicalfuture #robot #scifi | RoboCop (1987) Iron Man (2008)

If you want to hear true stories told in a unique way, search for The Moth on YouTube. This non–profit group dedicates itself to the art of storytelling. You might have amazing ideas or a great story, but telling it effectively takes certain skills. Here's an analogy: anyone can chronicle events ("This happened, and then… and then …"), but it takes a journalist who has studied journalistic skills to turn events into a story. You can think of storytelling as an art. That's what individuals who are invited to tell their stories in The Moth's podcasts discover.

Candidates undergo preliminary interviews to help them get the most out of their material. The process is similar to what presentation coaches do for TED events. I planned to tell the story of how I became a medical futurist from being a science fiction geek and physician. But the interviewer kept asking me about the dark future of technologies. At one point while showing me photos on her phone of people with implanted devices, she asked what makes someone a cyborg. I refrained from telling her that her smartphone basically made her a cyborg too. That smartphone with all its components, Internet connection and applications already augmented her capabilities functioning like an external brain.

A cyborg has organic and biomechatronic compounds. The latter includes the aspects of biology, mechanics and electronics. It has to be attached to or implanted into the human body though. It was an advance in human evolution when we went from stone tools to iron ones, and then to the wheel. Technology helped us evolve and get better at adapting to the changing environment.

Today it is the same but it takes place much faster. Cochlear implants, pacemakers and retinal implants seem and sound cybernetic, but these just help us live more normal lives. I don't see any problem with using devices to live healthier. There is a difference, though, when we start using them to augment human capabilities.

The ability of someone being able to afford a brain implant or exoskeleton, while another cannot, will create a new eco–system. Financial differences will lead to biological ones. Society must debate the ethical ramifications. Regulations must be established to prevent a single–minded focus on improving ourselves technologically.

It is possible that brain implants will improve memory and cognition. Implanted magnetic or RFID chips in our fingertip could replace passwords and house keys. Exoskeletons may boost our strength and let us run faster or jump higher. Already, there are cyborgs among us. Let me share some of their stories.

Jesse Sullivan became a cyborg when he was equipped with a bionic limb that was connected via nerve–muscle grafting. Aside from motor control over the limb by using his mind he can also feel temperature and pressure as he applies his grip.

Nigel Ackland lost part of his arm in a work accident. His new arm has a prosthetic hand that he controls via muscle movements in his intact forearm. The range of movement he can execute is extraordinary. He can move each of the five fingers independently to grip delicate objects or pour liquid into a glass.

Cameron Clapp was only 14 when he collapsed alongside a railroad track. The passing train severed both legs and an arm. His prosthetic legs are controlled by his brainwaves with the help of a microprocessor. Since his accident he has become both an athlete and an amputee activist.

Some people have deliberately chosen to become cyborgs. Neil Harbisson is an artist born with achromatopsia, a lack of color vision that leaves him seeing only shades of black–and–white. He has been fitted with an electronic eye that renders colors as musical sounds that let him hear color. He is now capable of experiencing colors beyond the scope of normal human perception.

Jerry Jalava lost a finger in a motorcycle accident, and decided to have a 2GB USB port embedded into his prosthesis. It obviously doesn't upload anything directly into his brain. One of, if not, the first cyborgs is Professor Steve Mann who designed a headset outfitted with a number of small computers and he can record and play video and audio through that.

It's straightforward to become a cyborg today. Web shops offer sterile implantable RFID chips and anyone can get theirs by going through a short procedure. But where is the limit? What is the threshold for becoming a cyborg? Should anyone be allowed to upgrade himself? Suppose hackers design their own interfaces–what then? These issues raise more questions than answers.

The movie *Transcendence* depicted a world with protests against cyborgs and overall technology. Such activist groups may be inevitable. But what is going to be their threshold? Professor Mann was kicked out of a McDonald's restaurant in Paris for wearing his headset which is attached to his head and thus cannot be removed without tools. The cashier thought he was deliberately filming employees for some nefarious purpose.

Years ago, people were stopped by the police because they were making a mobile phone call. Texting while driving is now the top cause of death among teenagers, surpassing drinking and driving. Overall, texting is involved in 25% of all car accidents in the US. Drivers were stopped and fined for using their Apple Watch while driving. Google Glass, digital contact lenses, and more devices are joining the line of distractions.

This distraction from ourselves is a huge challenge. Self–reflection is important in developing our personality and should be an essential part of our ego. Yet it only takes place when we are alone with our thoughts without the constant beeping and screen flashing of our smartphones. As technology plays a bigger and bigger role in our lives we might lose the chance to improve ourselves. My geek self wants to think that technology is the answer for everything, while my doctor self reminds me that we need to remain human. The solution may lie somewhere in the middle.

I don't doubt that as people discover how technology can improve their lives, the percentage of actual cyborgs in the society is going to mount. How society will look upon them will depend on the first crop that catches the media's attention. In the 2014 music video by Viktoria Modesta, the world's first amputee pop artist, she shows off her high–tech prosthetic leg. It creates an image more of a cyborg than of a disabled person.

Stelios Arcadiou, known as Stelarc, is a performance artist who believes that the human body is obsolete. In an attempt to prove so he had an artificial ear surgically attached to his forearm with the goal of implanting a microphone in it later. In another show he attached electrodes to himself so that people could activate his muscles through the Web.

Diversity isn't only about race, gender, and sexual orientation. It may have to include cyborgization as well. New laws might have to protect cyborgs from discrimination in work or in their personal lives. While race, gender, and orientation are not matters of choice, becoming a cyborg will be. The safety of implants and the ethical issues of living with such technologies may divide society. If and when it does we might lose the chance of upgrading ourselves in a way that keeps our humanity dominant.

Hopefully cyborg individuals and the culture behind upgrading will lead us in the right directions. Adding tech to our body should not be about fun or fashion. It is about quality of life for many. What makes someone a cyborg depends on the approach we take about it.

As long as we can keep the end product human it will be fine. We need to distinguish making oneself a cyborg on purpose versus welcoming technologies that improve well-being. I don't plan to implant an electronic eye any time soon, but if I were rendered blind, I might do anything to see again. Doing so would not make me less human. It would make me more.

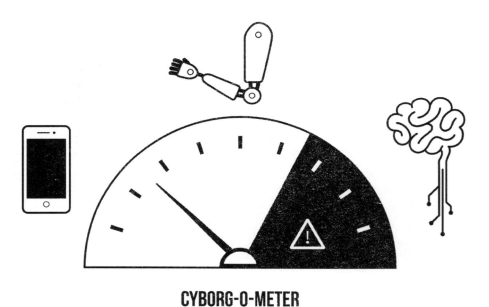

CYBORG-O-METER

WHAT IS THE SECRET TO A LONG LIFE?

#longevity #ageing | The Fountain (2006)

The World Congress of Gerontology and Geriatrics is a huge event attracting thousands of attendees and exhibitors. It is devoted to the field of ageing from a life sciences perspective to that of technology that can help the elderly live better. During one congress in Paris, a Frenchman in his seventies who was remarkably fit asked what the secret to a long life was. I thought I should ask him.

His question has been asked since time immemorial. The answer still isn't clear, but we may have come closer to answering it given the recent decades of research on ageing. Recent history has recorded individuals who have been documented to live more than 100 years. Such centenarians have surprisingly indulged in red wine, cigarettes, and red meat. At least one–third of our lifespan is influenced by our genetic background. The remainder involves lifestyle, exercise, and other factors. One way to weigh the contributions is to observe individuals over time.

In Alameda County, Californian residents filled out questionnaires once every decade between 1965 and 1999. The study concluded that healthier, longer lives were sustained by sleeping 7 to 8 hours a night, not smoking, exercising regularly, maintaining a desirable weight, and limiting the consumption of alcohol. These are generally known factors for a healthy life.

But people like to look at it from a less scientific point of view. The ending of the Monty Python movie, *The Meaning of Life*, says „Try to be nice to people, avoid eating fat, read a good book every now and then, get some walking in, and try and live together in peace and harmony with people of all creeds and nations." While it is hard not to concur, notable research has produced more complex suggestions about how to make longevity possible for everyone.

The ongoing Okinawa Centenarian Study in Japan analyzed hundred centenarians, their siblings, and a cohort of controls. At 81 years, life expectancy in the Okinawa prefecture is higher than the Japanese average. Aside from the beneficial effects of the Japanese lifestyle, diet, and regular exercise, the study teased out the genetic factors involved.

The Archon Genomics XPrize offered by the X Prize Foundation challenged participants to sequence the genomes of hundred centenarians. The point was to find what genetic differences, if any, existed between these older citizens and the rest of the population. The study collected samples from more than a hundred centenarians from around the world and made sequence data available to the public. The study came to an end in 2013 because subsequent developments had outpaced them. There is no single gene that contributes to extreme longevity.

Biological limitations might exist for how long someone can theoretically live. Presently 125 years is considered the upward limit. And yet gerontologists such as Aubrey de Grey claim that we can reverse ageing. His project has analyzed several aspects of ageing, from cancer types to normal cell death. A great deal of his research budget came from individual donors de Grey himself and Peter Thiel, Internet entrepreneur.

I bumped into a crowdfunding project called the Longevity Cookbook. It aims at creating guidelines about what diet can best promote longevity. Maria Konovalenko, a PhD student in ageing research who is behind this idea, thinks that the cure for ageing is already in its initial stages and exists in pharmacies. About forty existing drugs can extend the lifespan in laboratory animals. Evidence suggests that a combination of these may be able to extend human life, although side effects may be unavoidable. It would be necessary to carry out pre–clinical and clinical studies to identify appropriate doses and combinations of these drugs such as metformin, acetylcysteine or vitamin B6.

Konovalenko also mentioned the potential of gene therapy to halt ageing. Several dozen genes are known to be associated with longevity through animal studies. One strategy might be to pick the twenty most promising ones and inject them to old mice. We could identify any that bestowed the mice benefit and then test combinations for gene therapies intended for humans.

Other approaches to ageing include tissue engineering of solid organs and therapeutic cloning. In general terms the scientific community knows what to do. The question that remains is how we can accelerate research. The secret to long life may hinge on finding a way to apply big data to social information. We will have to create tools for mobilizing people and resources to counter ageing. Any approach towards ageing should be developed as an open project, such as the Genome Project or the Large Hadron Collider, otherwise research groups can hardly combine their efforts.

In 2013 Google spun off Calico that specialized in longevity research. Its modest mission statement speaks of "curing death" and every disease associated with ageing. Even if it sounds ambitious, what if their approach is the right one? Chronic diseases arise and are best treated individually. But what if ageing is the root cause of such conditions, and that by retarding ageing we also slow down the appearance of such diseases?

Knowledge about longevity continues to expand. But to what extent will we be able to live up to it? There might be drugs that extend life and technologies that aid the elderly. But if these do not become widely accessible society will divide into those who can afford to live longer and those who cannot.

When tissue engineering becomes commonplace, we might print out replacement organs. When technology can help people live better through either implanted microchips or attached devices, then we might redefine longevity from living longer to living better.

If ageing research keeps improving as it does, soon everyone will at least know what methods might help them live longer. Once basic health problems of underdeveloped regions are solved, the question will be not how to extend life but how society handles mentally and physically active centenarians having entirely different needs than the elderly today. The ultimate secret of long life then will be how to deal with it on the level of society.

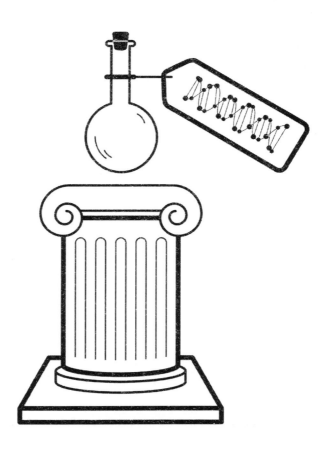

WHAT WOULD HAPPEN TO SOCIETY IF WE ALL LIVED BEYOND 130?

#longevity #medicalfuture #ageing | Metropolis (1927) Brazil (1985)

The Parliaments and Civil Society in Technology Assessment (PACITA) is a project of the European Union. By bringing stakeholders of healthcare together it hopes to design policy, gather technological solutions, and promote awareness of assisting an ageing society. I participated in one of its workshops at which we listened to possible scenarios and then had to come up with ideas about how to help society with technology. I enjoyed it very much. A key question was what would happen to society if we all lived beyond 130.

Life expectancy in classical Greece or Rome was 30 years. Starting in the 19th century it slowly changed. Since 1840, life expectancy at birth has risen about three months per year. This means that every year a newborn lives three months longer than those born the previous year. Sweden, which keeps exceptional demographic records, documents a female life expectancy of 45 in 1840 and 83 today.

Huge differences can of course exist between regions. Current life expectancy is 49 years in Swaziland and 83 in Japan. It is not obvious that people want to live longer. The Pew Research Center surveyed thousands of Americans in 2013. A third of them didn't want to live past the age of 80. Two–thirds didn't want to live past 90. Only a small minority of 8% wanted to live for more than a hundred years. Why don't people want to live longer?

Ageing is generally associated with deteriorating health and decrepitude. Ideally, this should improve first before life expectancy. The reality is that life expectancy improved so quickly in only a few decades that society hasn't been able to adjust. Some populations deal with this better than others. A prominent success is Japan.

In 2014 Japan had the highest proportion of elderly citizens. A third were more than 60, a quarter 65 or above, and 1 in 8 were 75 or above. Japanese companies are traditionally responsible for health insurance and regular medical check–ups for their employees. The Japanese are known to be disciplined and ready to implement lifestyle changes based on results.

Despite government policies for free childcare, or its emphasis on work–life balance, the Japanese contend with more chronic conditions than others. They will either have to raise retirement age to 75 or allow the influx of millions of immigrants by 2050 in order to have enough workers to support retirees.

If we look only at the effects of an ageing population, then extending lifespan will be devastating. More people will be dependent on worker generations who will have to pay higher taxes to provide care for their elders. But the point of longevity is not merely more years alive but an improvement in living those years.

Health economists should better explain how healthcare will change current economics. Linear thinking is out. People will live longer and in a probably good condition. Disruptive technologies will have a larger effect on the whole process than we see today. If innovations can't connect us better, then let's access care faster, or get personalized treatments if prevention is not enough. Society will adjust to new challenges.

Consider Alzheimer's and Parkinson's as examples within ageing populations. Technical solutions improve patient lives. Wright Stuff offers a range of products to make getting dressed easier for those who have lost the use of a hand. The company offers Dressing Sticks, a one–handed belt, sock aids, and even a one–handed nail clipper. Wearable cameras and augmented reality glasses can further help patients with Alzheimer's disease. These gadgets can snap hundreds of pictures a day from the user's perspective and thus log their lives. Tablet applications such as Speak For Yourself put vocabularies of 13,000 words within reach of a few touches on a screen. As sound quality improves, synthetic voices are becoming more natural sounding.

Even small ideas matter. A German senior center used the idea of fake bus stops to keep Alzheimer's patients from wandering off. Because short term memory has failed but long–term memory is fine, such patients know what the sign means, and they stop. It has been a huge success in Germany, and now other clinics want to use it. Devices could address fall prevention by transmitting an alert to a local clinic or hospital. GTX Corp came up with a smart shoe that helps individuals find their way home, and orientate themselves while walking down the street.

I asked Zoltan Istvan of the Transhumanist Party and Presidential candidate for the 2016 US elections for his views on this. If we live past 130 years, society will fundamentally change. We will have to contend with social welfare and retirement systems that cannot sustain themselves. We will have family issues too given that being married for a hundred years is different from being hitched for 50 years.

More importantly, if society can make it another 30 years then the age of indefinite life spans will be upon us. When that happens, social institutions will change dramatically because every decade that we progress new technologies will ensue. A few possibilities are growing organs outside the body, or ectogenesis, uploading individual minds to computers, and the voluntary elimination of genders.

Expanding life expectancy is a long–term task. If increasing numbers of people start living beyond 100, then the structure of society will change. Young workers will have to deal with the fact that people will retire increasingly later. Both will take place in coming decades. In the meantime, new technologies can transform how elderly people will live among their younger cohorts. Digital solutions should not push them to the periphery but keep them connected to the center.

When living beyond a hundred becomes a decision, rather than an opportunity, it is going to pose ethical issues to society it has never had before. There is a saying that the first person to live beyond 150 has already been born. If it is true, we might be the new generation of super–centenarians.

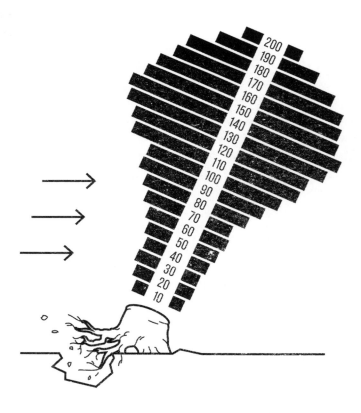

SHOULD I GET CRYOPRESERVED WHEN I DIE?

#longevity #cryonics #cryogenics I 2001: A Space Odyssey (1968) Alien (1979)

A serial entrepreneur and angel investor asked to have a coffee in order to talk about investments in future healthcare. He was about 80 and excited to show me how the contact list in his Blackberry worked. He asked tons of questions about where medical technology was heading, and I shared my ideas with him. He said he was a techie but curious about upcoming trends. At the end of our discussion he asked if he could pose a personal question: should he get cryopreserved when he died? Talking about death can be disconcerting aside from the fact that I don't provide advice on such a sensitive topic. He insisted, I relented, and he was not relieved.

Freezing someone after death in the hope of being awakened later is called cryopreservation. The field is called cryonics. Think of all the movies that depict it. After a long space flight, you wake up as if it were a typical Sunday morning. *Aliens, Avatar, Interstellar, and 2001: Space Odyssey* all involve such scenarios. In *Star Wars: The Empire Strikes Back*, Han Solo is famously frozen in carbonite–a prime example of cryopreservation. Solo woke up temporarily blind, but future patients will have to worry about more than that–such as never waking up again.

Let's consider other problems. Physical inactivity for a week leads to muscle atrophy and blood clots. Bacteria in our digestive system cannot survive prolonged temperature drops or lack of food. And yet these organisms are crucial to our health. Lungs in stasis become full of mucus, and the brain starts resembling that of Alzheimer patients.

When a person is declared dead, the Alcor Cryonics company leaps into action. The deceased who agreed to cryopreservation and has already paid for it, is placed on an ice bed that circulates cold water. Respiration is restored, and about sixteen medications are administered. Their aim is to maintain tissue viability for as long as possible. Technicians access the heart with various tubes, making it possible to replace blood with "vitrification fluid".

Vitrification may sound awful because it transforms a substance into glass. It aims to prevent organs and other tissues from irreversibly freezing. It has successfully been used to preserve human egg cells. A rabbit kidney was once froze using this liquid and then successfully transplanted into another rabbit after re–warming.

Stories about human hibernation are many. Although this one is without evidence, the British Medical Journal published an article about Russian farmers who were said to hibernate. When they sensed winter was approaching they entered a state of "chronic famine", gathered around the stove, and fell into a deep slumber. Who knows whether this tale is real?

In 1999 a Swedish radiologist, Anna Bagenholm, suffered a ski accident and lay trapped under a layer of ice for 80 minutes. After 40 minutes her circulation stopped. When she was found her temperature was 13.7 Celsius degrees, the lowest recorded. More than a hundred doctors worked on her, and eventually recovered nearly in full. Only nerve injury in her feet and hands persisted.

In emergencies there isn't always time to assess the patient's particulars and come up with the best solution. Surgeons, for example, fight against the clock. Others want to buy time by lowering body temperatures. Such approaches can save lives. Cooling the body sufficiently can put it in a state of suspended animation–without a pulse, breathing, or brain activity. For cryopreservation blood is replaced with ice–cold fluids that prevent tissue damage while keeping them functional. Successful trials have concluded in dogs. We now wait to transfer the method to injured patients.

Photos on wall of the Alcor Cryonics headquarters show people who are already cryopreserved and in stasis. They have about 120 patients and the number is growing even though there is no scientific evidence these people could ever be resuscitated. They rely on the hope that scientific progress will continue being exponential, and at some point resuscitation will be possible.

Ethical and legal issues around this are huge. In France, cryonics is not considered a legal mode of body disposal. In 1995 the American Cryonics Society asked Charles Tandy, Associate Professor of Humanities, to share his thoughts. Tandy cited four principles behind cryopreservation including respect for autonomy, the concept of not to do harm, to do beneficent acts, and social justice. He concluded that „biomedical professionals have a strong and actual obligation to help insure cryonic–hibernation of the cryonics patient". The Cryonics Institute currently has more than 1,300 members.

If I'm ready to pay for such a service, who has the right to stop me? If preservation technology becomes viable, how will resuscitated people integrate themselves back into society? If the technology is increasingly misunderstood, when is cryopreserved patient declared irreversibly dead? Cryogenics generates disturbing questions. It makes people concerned about the technological developments. Helping people understand potential uses can bridge the gap between their reality and the ethical bubble.

Transhumanists such as Zoltan Istvan are naturally optimistic. He thinks people who want to live indefinitely should get cryopreserved. He believes that it is just a matter of time before we discover technologies that can revive frozen people. He estimates that in 50 years we will have such technology, if not before. Preparing society for such an invention might be a bigger challenge than creating such a technology. We are not ready for either.

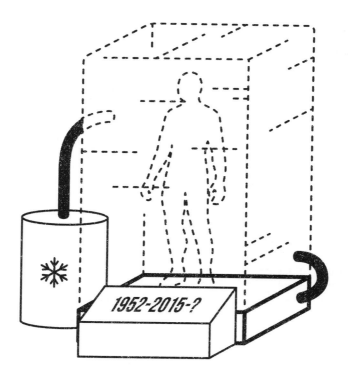

WILL NANOROBOTS SWIM IN OUR BLOODSTREAM?

#nanotech #medicalfuture #nanotechnology | *Fantastic Voyage (1966)*

The best thing about being a medical futurist is that you never know what doors will open for you. Sometimes I receive so many exciting inquiries for collaboration or other engagements that it energizes me for months. Recently, a science fiction writer approached me about a novel he was working on. He was writing a futuristic novel that featured technology that had not been invented yet or concepts we don't have to worry about yet either.

He was inspired by the novel *Diaspora* by Greg Egan which raised a number of issues about scientific methods and technological directions. We met, and as he poured out one idea after another my task was to find some scientific justification for them. I enjoyed it thoroughly.

His main character was a utopian cyborg that had numerous micro-chip and sensor implants. His cyborg wouldn't have to eat or drink because the tiny robots in his body would produce everything he needed. I suggested that these nanorobots might also heal tissues from inside, and bridge communication between his internal milieu and an external device. We bantered crazy ideas back and forth. When he wondered out loud whether nanorobots would ever live in our bloodstream in the future he seemed doubtful. But my answer brightened him up again.

Ray Kurzweil has mentioned robots on the nanometer scale –one billionth of a meter– many times. He has imagined us wearing a special belt containing a swarm of nanorobots. These nanobots could deliver the nutrients to the body in the needed amount. Eventually, such nanobots would replace our internal organs. Nanobots by 2020 could upload our minds to the cloud, creating a connection between our nervous system and earth–wide computing. This kind of futuristic scenario is the kind that might worry Transhumanists.

The concept is not new. The 1966 movie, *Fantastic Voyage* explored shrinking a medical team to microscopic size in order to save a renowned scientist's life. The Argonauts travel through the bloodstream into the brain where the crew uses a laser gun to blast away a blood clot. Now, how about a nanometer sized cage in real life that lets out insulin but doesn't get attacked by our immune system? Imagine this in diabetes, or the same approach for releasing dopamine directly to the brainstem in Parkinson's disease. Chemotherapy could likewise be injected into cancer cells while keeping healthy cells untouched. There are ongoing research projects for all these applications.

In 2014 the Max Planck Institute in Stuttgart, Germany announced that it had created scallop–like microbots designed to swim in bodily fluids such as blood or cerebrospinal fluid. Their shell is only a few times wider than the thickness of a human hair. Their size will soon get smaller and the microbots have additional functions.

The John Hopkins University has developed robots only one millimeter across that can take biopsies inside the colon. Patients swallow a tiny capsule, and the robotic biopsy comes out with it. Engineers are working on having these robots perform surgery inside the colon, too. We may be only years away from having actual working nanorobots.

The real advantage of having robots on the nanometer scale is having them work in large groups. One minuscule robot cannot make much of a difference. But a million of them can move a house. Scientists at SRI International, an American non–profit research institute, created such a swarm. The ant–like robots are controlled magnetically, are very fast, can locate and use tools. Moving through even flexible surfaces they can construct three–dimensional structures at an amazing pace. They could revolutionize both biotechnology and electronics manufacturing.

Other inventions include a DNA box with proteins that induce cell death; it opens only in proximity to cancer cells. Another nanocage developed at Oxford University can potentially deliver drugs directly inside specific cells. The cage prevents DNA inside it from being destroyed by enzymes, even after days. Using nanorobots could eliminate side effects from cancer treatments, thus solving one of the biggest issues in chemotherapy treatment because only cancer cells are targeted. In the future the nanobots could be administered by simple injection, a skin patch, or merely swallowing a liquid.

A favorable sign regarding these developments is the entrance of the pharmaceutical giant Pfizer into the field. A partner lab is producing innovative DNA molecules that can be programmed to reach specific targets or perform surgery. They could be powered via existing chemicals in the blood, or by internal or external sources. These latter issues have not yet been solved, but there is no reason to believe that they won't be.

The question is not whether nanorobots will swim in our bloodstream but to what extent we will let this happen. If authorities fail to anticipate potential dangers and educate the public about them, society will resist such techniques given that movies typically depict such inventions as evil ways to control innocent people. *Transcendence (2014)*, ineffectively, illustrates such a backlash.

Might there come a point at which the overlap between nanorobots and our own cells—organic material merging with synthetic ones—becomes problematic? That is, if nanobots can replace cell functions or even the entire cell, then what part of us remains human? We already know that neurons can live in harmony with a biochip and make connections with electrodes. What happens when we and the tiny computers living inside us become one? Do we want to become one in this way? Are there more advantages than risks to nanotechnology? The word symptom might be erased from our vocabulary when nobody uses it any longer. If nanobots alerted us to imminent illnesses before the disease actually developed, then we would never experience a symptom again.

In this way nanobots might become more effective at fighting microbes than our own immune system. Nanobots in our central nervous system might boost our intelligence or link us up with computers as depicted in *The Matrix.* The coming years in medicine will not face these issues. Instead, we will have to face the legal boundaries when nanobots first go to clinical trial. We will see headlines warning of threats and dangers to society. But if we can treat cancer more precisely, and be warned about diseases that are likely to develop in us, then I am ready to take the risk.

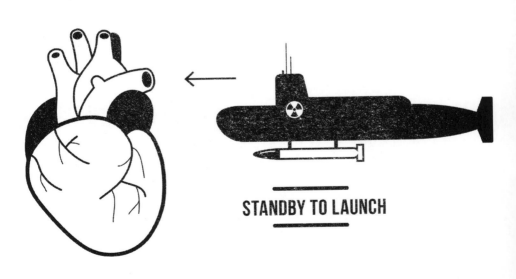

STANDBY TO LAUNCH

WHY ARE FUTURISTS USUALLY WRONG ABOUT HEALTHCARE?

#futurism #medicalfuture I The Congress (2013)

Not everyone is pleased hearing some of my radical views about the future of medicine. Some might ask hard questions or make sarcastic remarks. It also happened during an interview.

Interviewers tend to be objective. They like to discover this field for themselves and ask questions that lead to vibrant discussions. I once had an interview with a journalist who was eager to learn more. She brought up the singularity, transhumanism, and many philosophies. Yet she seemed skeptical about it all, and kept raising controversial questions. I began to feel that she wanted to goad me into admitting the dangers and threats of new technologies. Our whole conversation came to a point when she asked why futurists like me are always wrong in their predictions.

Personally, she was set against most technology. After enduring a barrage of her negativity I asked about the reason behind her attitude. She said that technology was categorically bad. She blamed futurists for never preparing people for what was coming next even though predicting the future as their job. I immediately understood her problem: she didn't know what futurists do.

Futurists or futurologists systematically explore possibilities in any area ranging from energy and healthcare to defense and finance. They try to predict how these trends could come about and then change in the future so that people affected by those fields can prepare.

The biggest proportion of futurists today work as consultants or speakers. Jules Verne, H.G. Wells, and other authors could be considered futurists: they had an ability to explore details that nobody had pondered before and come up with ideas no one had thought of. This aptitude draws on skills taken from problem solving, planning, computer science, and psychology.

Merely thinking about the future is not futurism. Giving people directions so they prepare themselves for change is. Despite this, most of the people I meet want to know about predictions and dates as soon as they discover that I'm a medical futurist.

I asked Ian Pearson, futurist author of *You Tomorrow*, about his take on this. He said that the most important skill is systems thinking. Given that many factors will affect what happens next, and when, it is an asset to think about the big picture and visualize how things interact. Doing so is different from everyday thinking that often becomes too focused on tiny details while ignoring outside forces. If you ignore such forces, you introduce error. Being precise about only a few of these is counterproductive if you ignore other factors that might be larger. It is more important to take them in the big picture and include all the influences you can think of. Even if you lack accurate figures, you can allow for effects by subjective estimates. You won't always be able to give an accurate prediction, but at least you'll have a good idea what the likely margins of error might be or where the branch points for alternative scenarios might occur.

Ray Kurzweil is famous for his predictions and the accuracy he claims. A Wikipedia entry is dedicated to all the predictions he has made in his books. By 2022, he says, medical technology will be more than a thousand times advanced compared to today. In the 2020s medical nanobots will perform detailed brain scans on live patients. By 2099 the concept of "life expectancy" will become irrelevant thanks to medical immortality and advanced computation. Critics object that his predictions come with so many loopholes that they verge on being unfalsifiable.

In 2010 TIME magazine complained that teleportation, flying cars, jet packs, meals in pills, and cyborg abilities have not become reality by the 2010s. Wild and careless predictions not only confuse people, but can also scare them. Social media illustrates a perfect forum for over– and under–estimating important trends. News sites using link baiting (the practice of creating spectacular titles with the aim of people clicking on them) can easily make people attend to something while other trends with bad marketing can fall behind. The latter are particularly hard to unearth.

This is why futurists, compared to laypeople, use different methods when they think about future trends. They shape potential scenarios depending on whether they want to know how people might adopt to, what economic benefits it might bring. They can scour other industries for relevant technologies, organize workshops with experts, or create plausible roadmaps for a given technology. Futurists usually have a wide field of methods to pick from, but when it comes to healthcare that field turns to thin ice. Predicting the future is easy. Making it right is hard.

Medicine is full of ethical, legal, safety, social, and political landmines. It is evidence–based, meaning that studies must prove that a method or a drug is actually efficient. These must be safe given that lives are at stake. Compared to other industries healthcare regulation is strict and expensive.

The biggest difference between healthcare and other industries is the difficulty with which technological improvements are implemented in practice. If someone invented a fully functional nanocage that could deliver drugs to specific cells, it wouldn't be available tomorrow. It might take a decade to wind its way through the regulatory process and necessary clinical trials before being approved–if at all.

I don't think that developing healthcare products is fundamentally slow. But the methods we have are. With cognitive computers that analyze big data sets and draw conclusions, it should get better. Using social media channels, today's futurists can connect to millions of people and gather the best pieces of information if they have digital skills required for digesting them. Being a futurist today means surfing the waves of change instead of coming up with static future scenarios. Experts, key information, and the people who predict future trends are now scattered around the world. Digital tools could bring them together.

What we could learn in the past decades is that predicting the exact dates when big technologies become available doesn't help. Whether these predictions are very accurate or miserably fail, no stakeholder of healthcare could have used these to make steps forward in designing a better care system. What can help them though are clear directions and suggestions about what to do next.

Healthcare will only get better if individuals understand the need to change their own lives and themselves. If this happens, the healthcare system will follow their lead. Responsible futurists must make sure that these directions are safe and valid. We will be wrong sometimes, but we can't prepare for the weather unless we look out often. And someone needs to keep that window clean.

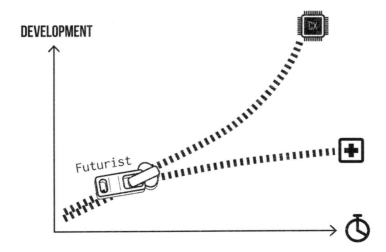

SHOULD WE BE AFRAID OF ARTIFICIAL INTELLIGENCE IN MEDICINE?

#artificialintelligence #ai #deeplearning #machinelearning
Forbidden Planet (1956)

What I enjoy most about my job is being in contact with people around the world. Some are global experts while others are simply interested in the future of medicine. Through social media I can monitor what they talk about, and I question them. Being in touch is the prime time of my work.

Since the publication of my earlier book *The Guide to the Future of Medicine*, I have received countless messages through my website and social media. On "The Medical Futurist" Facebook page, I share key announcements about the future of medicine every day. Interestingly, when I share my thoughts about artificial intelligence, my followers tend to get engaged. They ask whether we should be afraid of it. In a nutshell, we should. But not yet.

Supercomputers depend on brute force. Cognitive computers are a matter of algorithms. Artificial intelligence is yet again different. It means that computers should be able to analyze problems and solve them even with methods they have never seen before. After all, that's what humans do. Our flexibility is our greatest strength. It is what makes our nervous system one of the best inventions of the universe. It might be a part of our evolution to design intelligent machines and let them improve at their own pace. Or doing so might be the end of the human era.

Elon Musk, Stephen Hawking, and many others have voiced their fears about artificial intelligence. By definition, truly artificial intelligence would be able to improve itself at a pace that our brains cannot match, thus overshadowing us and deciding our fate. We might not be needed any longer. We might merely be consuming energy that machines could use to keep improving themselves. This impasse is not about computers being evil, but about each side's basic needs. If you read the most thoughtful books on this topic, you will see that it is a plausible scenario. Examples include *Superintelligence* by Bostrom, or *Our Final Invention* by Barrat.

The Turing test determines whether an algorithm is artificially intelligent. It has received some criticism lately, but most computer scientists still consider it the right approach. I once had a discussion with a chat bot claimed to have passed the Turing test. It took only a few minutes to satisfy myself that it was just an algorithm. That's how bad it was in conversation. I asked how many apples John has if he has four times more than Amy, who has two and a half. In return the chat bot asked if we really wanted to talk about apples.

When I tried to move the discussion forward it became stuck and repetitive, and that was it. An algorithm may beat the best chess players in the world, but it cannot answer a simple question. Computers are amazing at specific tasks. The challenge comes when their capabilities need to resemble ours.

There is Artificial Narrow Intelligence, which today you can find in your car, smartphone, spam filter, Google Translate, Facebook, Amazon, Google, and many more places. The world's best chess, scrabble, and backgammon players are now all such systems. Next is sophistication known as Artificial General Intelligence, which has some ability to reason, plan, solve problems, think abstractly, and come up with complex ideas. Finally, there is Artificial Superintelligence, which will be smarter than the best human brains. This is the evolution ahead of us. The steps between these three stages require refined developments, and so it won't happen tomorrow.

Narrowing down possible AI scenarios to negative and positive ones simplifies the issue. On the positive side, AI changes life for the better. It will plan ahead so we get the best out of all circumstances. It will talk with us and help us make advantageous decisions. It can bring about economic equality because it will better know how to share goods and resources among populations. It will design new devices and technologies for us because its primary goal is to assist humans. It sounds like the first part of a movie that shows a utopia just before everything goes berserk.

The negative side maintains that we can't create AI in a way that makes it friendly. It will see that we consume energy that they could use themselves. They might destroy or enslave us as a result. AI will know more, weigh decisions better, and eventually control our individual lives. Remember *The Matrix*?

Both these scenarios can be applied to medicine. AI could organize the entire healthcare system for the benefit of patients, physicians, and researchers, even hospital administrators. It could calculate patient risk based on personal data obtain from all our devices. Because it knows our genomics background, family history, and blood tests, it could inform us of its decisions about lifestyle changes we must make, and it would raise our fees accordingly because doing so we benefit society as a whole.

For physicians, AI would handle administration, help with difficult decisions, and keep them perfectly up–to–date. Their job would be reduced to keeping in touch with patients who choose to get treatment from a person instead of an AI. If an algorithm can improve a chess player, it can improve what a physician does as well. It doesn't have to be a replacement, but merely an aid. The stethoscope transformed medical practice in the 19th century. AI can be the stethoscope of the 21st century if we can make it friendly.

With AI medical research would become real–time, data–based, and essentially limitless. Software in the Internet of Things would analyze, diagnose, and dictate treatment based on changes in patient lifestyle or health status. Epidemics would not occur because AI would spot and isolate the first cases before they exploded in a chain reaction.

While many of these considerations don't involve people, I think most of them are still quite favorable. If an AI can solve one's health problems, provide empathy, and conduct ongoing research then who would complain that they are not part of the process? I remain confident that we can deliberately transform healthcare by working together with AI.

The negative scenario removes us from decision–making. When AI always knows better, we are reduced to puppets. Both scenarios can coexist, and we need ethical debates and regulations concerning where AI is needed and where it is not. It is more likely now that AI will not be friendly, but we have only taken small steps to address this. With proper regulations we might not end up with an AI that came out of someone's garage and which we cannot control. AI could and should be humanity's greatest invention. We should celebrate as we gradually watch it improve in a way we are happy about it.

While AI poses threat to society, medicine may not be the area most affected. Many aspects of healthcare could be revolutionized by AI without it putting lives at risk or physician jobs in jeopardy. AI is being developed not to replace the stakeholders in medicine, but to provide them with care they have never received before.

Cognitive computers such as IBM's Watson and Synapse will be in the forefront for the next few years. Be prepared for headlines about better algorithms that drive cars more safely and efficiently than people can; oversee the financial world; or pick new football players in drafts by equalizing the advantages among teams. When experts finally put aside the Turing test and design a better one, there might not be a definitive line between human and artificial intelligence any longer. That juncture will make it harder to appreciate that artificial intelligence has finally here.

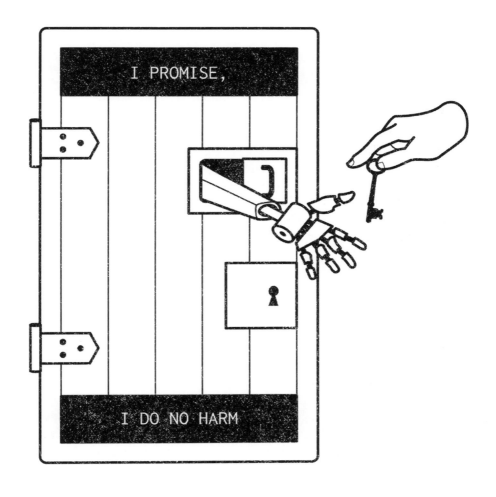

HOW DOES TECHNOLOGY CHANGE SEXUALITY?

#medicalfuture #sexuality | A.I. Artificial Intelligence (2001)
The Zero Theorem (2013)

At the first e–health conference in Melbourne, a nice group chatting at the bar dropped a bomb by asking how technology would change sexuality. Such a question deserved a colorful answer.

Many movies have tried to suggest what the future of sex would look like. *Logan's Run* in 1976 describes a hedonistic life in awful attire. *A.I.: Artificial Intelligence* in 2001 featured Jude Law as Gigolo, a male prostitute robot called Mecha programmed to mimic love. *In Her (2013)*, the main character had virtual sex with an AI operating system. *Ex Machina (2015)* made us squeamish about falling in love with a robot. These movies all used some kind of technology in depicting the future of sex. Is it really the future?

Virtual reality can potentially have an influence on sex. Early in 2015 in Los Angeles an application for the Oculus Rift virtual reality headset was demonstrated at a conference dedicated to sex and technology. The Red Light Center ushered people into a virtual night club where they watched virtual people. This was only the beginning, the company said. They plan to let people have sex with adult film entertainers in a virtual realm. They also plan to connect people this way by using adult toys. The original idea addressed couples in long–distance relationships, but a clamor for virtual sex by potential users prompted them to expand the options offered. One audience consists of military spouses doing their duties overseas.

Sexting is a new word in our vocabulary. It stands for sexual communication with another person through digital devices. Using virtual reality headsets for this purpose is a no–brainer. If you think doing so entirely removes the most important element of human touch from relationships, let me raise the stakes.

With properly augmented reality devices we will project digital pictures onto real life sceneries. People might buy apps that project their favorite movie stars onto real people, or create scenes they could never experience in real life. Whether it sounds awful or not, those trying virtual or augmented reality understand the power of this technology. Companies are also working on printing out virtual odors. Stars could sell their natural odor or perfume to influence the end user's pheromones.

The Hug Shirt allows people to send hugs over distance, just like a text message. The Bluetooth shirt has sensors and actuators, and is connected to a smartphone app. It can feel the strength, duration, and location of the touch, skin warmth, and the heart rate of the sender. The actuators then recreate the same touch sensation on the shirt worn by the distant loved one.

I still cannot decide whether Kiss Transmission is real or just a joke, but a 2011 video shows how a French kiss can be sent wirelessly to loved ones. Alternatively, the developer says that celebrity kisses could be purchased and shared by users. This is a direction perhaps no emotionally healthy person wants.

When Apple announced new features of its iOS in 2015, one called reproductive health tracking made the news. The iPhone would now let people track exactly how often and in what way they engage in sex. Users click on the Sexual Activity feature, enter information about date, time or using protection. Users see their sexual activities over time plotted on colorful graphs.

Some of the more exotic options might create an unwanted picture of the future of sexuality. But let's consider those living in distant relationships, or those who just can't find their place in society and struggle to find intimate relationships. As the global population continues to grow, social anxiety becomes more prevalent and the pressure on people to find love builds, making technology more needed to improve or at least supply some form of human touch.

Technosexuals such as Davecat live with "synthetic" partners, life sized dolls. He says he felt isolated and alone, without a place in society. After he began his relationship with his synthetic wives, everything changed. He says he is happy now and that his friends accept his choice. He told me he needed his dolls to start living a better life and that he's less sad than he was living alone. While I understand people's reaction to his viewpoint, it's hard to argue with his last point.

Japanese companies are currently working on robots with which users can have intercourse. If such robots can mimic that satisfactorily, perhaps those who struggle with forming real–life relationships will opt for them. Some robots such as the silicone–and–metal TrueCompanion can sense the user's movements and voice, and respond accordingly. It costs thousands of dollars, but a low–budget alternative is also available that has no arms or legs and can't talk about anything besides sexual acts. The male version is slightly cheaper. The RealDoll company manufactures adult dolls equipped with artificial intelligence that, the company claims, can substitute for real–life conversations.

Out of all these inventions, teledildonics is one of the most unconventional I have ever encountered. It represents the development of automated sex toys that are controlled either by a remote user or by a program. I can see future headlines about lawsuits following accidents during intercourse with robots. One cannot yet see the effect these inventions will have on society as a whole. They might make people less lonely in this harsh and complicated world. But if the human touch vanishes because there is no need for it anymore, it might bring about a new generation that can pleasure itself but not understand the meaning of love.

I have saved the most extreme example for last. I mentioned that optogenetics can activate specific neural cells with a particular wavelength of light. If our cells become engineered with this capacity, special lights can create the feeling of caress, and orgasm. Imagine future sex robots with LEDs all over their bodies flashing lights in programmed patterns downloadable through your smartphone app.

Self–Stimulation Addiction might receive its own code in the International Statistical Classification of Diseases in the future. If a microchip with the ability to trigger feelings of extreme pleasure on demand is ever developed, some people will lack the willpower to use it only on a selective basis.

If there is significant demand for this, the industry will boom. Obviously I belong to the skeptics about this. The Transhumanist Zoltan Istvan told me the question is not how technology changes sexuality, but whether sexuality can survive technology. He doesn't think it will. Sexuality, like all social rituals, is something that will not be needed in a world where offspring are born in a test tube, or even where the idea of having offspring is abandoned altogether.

This picture will probably disturb many people, but if technological solutions help people solve their need to connect, demand will lead to a swarm of high–tech products. The challenge will not be to decide whether they are good or bad, but to make sure that people will still understand, and what is more important, require the human touch in their relationships.

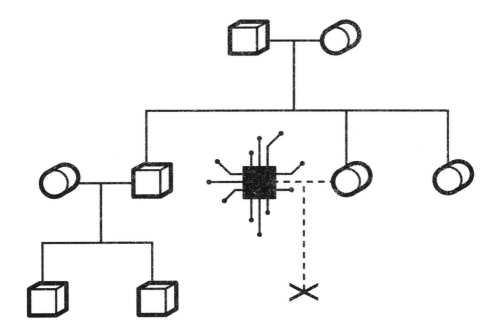

WHAT IF PEOPLE WANT TO REPLACE HEALTHY BODY PARTS FOR PROSTHETICS?

#medicalfuture #digitalhealth #ethics | Blade Runner (1982)

My medical school in Budapest was named after Ignaz Semmelweis, the "savior of mothers", who introduced the practice of washing hands with chlorinated water in 1847. Before that, doctors moved between the pathology and the obstetrics departments without washing their hands. This led to childbed fever, a common and often fatal infection. The notion of constantly improving the practice of medicine is still part of the university's approach.

Recently I was invited to an ethics debate in which mostly psychologists and social scientists participated. They asked me to speak about the most mind–blowing examples of future medical technology so that they could discuss their ethical implications. The discussion was quite heated.

I felt that they wanted to challenge my optimistic views about medicine's future. One panelist asked what would happen to society if people started asking for prosthetic devices even though they were healthy. She meant what would happen if augmenting the human body becomes technically possible while ethically impermissible.

If printing out organs becomes possible, beauty clinics will provide not only Botox treatments and skin rejuvenators, but new organs as well. When a prosthetic hand becomes sophisticated, flexible, and cool, healthy people will be ready to give up their healthy appendages for those. Perhaps if exoskeletons are cheap and comfortable and augment normal human capabilities, people will be more reckless and not worry about having an accident.

The future depends on three legs: how technology becomes affordable and efficient, being prepared for this by acquiring skills in digital literacy, and forming a bridge between the two. If any of these fail we will fail as a society. This is a highly simplified point of view, but it underscores the notion that it's going to be challenging. If technology is amazing but we cannot use it as we should, then we will have a technocracy in which tech skills are more important than anything else. If we upgrade ourselves but technology remains a commodity for only the wealthy, that is going lead us into chaos.

New responsibilities come with waves of change. When I decide to buy a wearable device to measure my sleep quality it doesn't entail any risk. I can put it down and never use it again. But if the technology I opt for must be irreversibly attached or implanted, that is a different issue. There will be a point at which we are more cyborg than biologically human. Groups of bioethicists try to define that point, but it will still vary among groups of people. Everyone must be able to decide for themselves, but this assumes that people are capable of making such decisions. Are they?

Matthew James was born with dysmelia, a congenital disorder causing deformed limbs. When he was 14 years–old, James told his favorite Formula One team, Mercedes, that he would display their logo on his prosthesis if they would support him financially. He received £30,000, but Mercedes did not take up on his offer for advertising space. The story shows that the implementation of such innovations in the everyday lives cannot depend purely on individual entrepreneurship.

The Alternative Limb Project started in 2011 thanks to the prosthetic limb designer Sophie De Oliveira Barata. She was inspired when her youngest client, who had lost a leg at the age of 2, asked Sophie to design a personalized and realistic leg for her. Patients can choose prosthetics in different styles and made from materials such as porcelain, steam punk, feather, crystal, or spike. They can pay for the device out of pocket, or through a sponsor or employer. While the project represents a good cause, people with intact limbs might start asking for these alternative prosthetics because it could help them express themselves artistically.

Today, society struggles to fight gender, racial, sexual and financial inequality. Future people may make themselves smarter, faster, and healthier only by virtue of being able to afford them. How would we prepare society for the time when financial differences lead to biological ones? Should anyone control this or will we let capitalism do it? One sounds worse than the other. Individuals will not have the required knowledge about high–tech technologies to determine how they will influence the public with their decisions. And capitalism will certainly not provide the most desirable outcomes when it comes to health.

A biotechnology black market also looms in the future. Printed prosthetics, sensors, brain microchips, biomaterials, and artificial tissues will be available through the same methods that today's startups take advantage of. While companies will have to comply with numerous rules and regulations, the black market will focus solely on providing devastated people in need with solutions. Avoiding all rules and guidelines means a huge risk for failure, data privacy, and ethical issues.

If a patient knows there is a technological solution for their health problem, but has no access to it, they will keep on going until they do. This might be the worst issue of all. Sterile, implantable RFID devices are available on the Web; many people have already got them implanted by tattoo artists so that they can open smartphone apps or garage doors with their hands. Given that there are no regulations for this at present, there is no a way to prevent people from implanting these chips. We simply haven't given the issue much thought yet.

Consider another scenario involving technology that extends life past its natural term. A grandmother in the US had had a stroke, but her pacemaker kept her alive. It was illegal to turn off the pacemaker. And so her body was not allowed to die even though her brain already had. The impasse led to financial disaster for the family. There are similar reports about people living with pacemakers who suffer a lot from the electrical shocks the pacemaker automatically delivers while a person is dying. Such complications have led experts to suggest preemptively shutting down pacemakers when a patient's end is near.

Today, the milestones of birth and death are quite clear. With technologies that can give us a chance for better and longer lives, these milestones may also be challenged. What shall we do and who shall intervene when the brain is dead but the body is kept alive by implanted devices? Augmenting our physical and cognitive capabilities to almost no limits, or extending our lives to well over 100 will lead to questions we don't have any answers for.

Office workers can augment their capabilities by drinking coffee. Certain athletes use illicit drugs and biological methods such as influencing gene expression of certain genes to augment themselves despite the practice being prohibited. Who is going to stop me from buying a thin exoskeleton for my legs so I can run faster? Suppose I use legal cognitive drugs to improve my performance instead of coffee? What if I can choose the genetic features of my baby's DNA? Genetically engineering future children or even ourselves might become possible with the advances of genome sequencing and DIY biotechnology.

Ever–improving technologies open up a lot of ethical challenges. Most people I talk to think that is a reason good enough to avoid the tech revolution. This is a reason why having ethical debates will be more important than ever, and their outcome should reach people worldwide, something social media can facilitate. If the fear and risks had made us slow down the development of existing technology, we might have never had cars, pharmaceuticals, or computers.

We need to take big risks now. Otherwise healthcare will never be affordable and efficient. If we, as individuals, can prepare in time, there is a chance. If groups of bioethicists can help us prepare, the likelihood of success becomes much bigger. If we start discussing all the potential advantages and problems at home, at work, and on a societal level, the chance becomes bright. I hope people will be willing to take these risks if the end of the tunnel is marked by healthier lives.

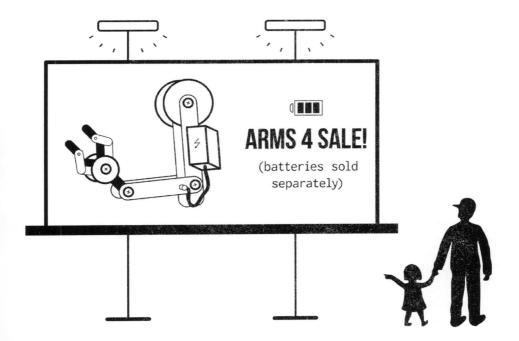

HOW CAN WE PREVENT BIOTERRORISM FROM HIJACKING INNOVATIONS?

#medicalfuture #bioterrorism #ethics I Transcendence (2014)

When Marx Goodman, author of *Future Crimes*, spoke in Silicon Valley, he painted a highly negative future in which technology empowered criminals. There was a lively discussion that brought up the issue of bioterrorism. When I gave a keynote at the Interactive Cologne Festival about what the future holds for us, I thought there would be questions about wearables and health management, but an engineering student was very curious about bioterrorism.

In the US the health records of more than 100 million citizens have been breached. In early 2015, Anthem Blue Cross notified 80 million members that their records had been compromised in a cyber attack. If so many patients' medical data are not secure, the gigantic amount of data generated by the patients themselves with home devices will be in worse situation.

We share far more information about ourselves than we think we do. Check mypermissions.org to see what services and apps you have already allowed to access your personal information. Wearable devices coming from startups all over the world measure and store data. End users can only hope they are secure.

It has been shown many times that medical devices such as pacemakers or insulin pumps can be hacked over the web. Security experts have warned that someone could be murdered this way. How can we prevent wearable devices connected to our physiology from being hacked and controlled remotely?

Company by company, development cannot ensure this. Authorities and governments should take precautions and be proactive–except they don't and they aren't. Medical equipment software was designed decades ago without security in mind, and now we are paying the price for lack of foresight. In June 2015, Chinese hackers infected devices in the radiology department of a European hospital that let hackers roam hospital network, and sent the gathered data to China.

Physicians worry now when patients Google their symptoms and treatments, and bring misinformation they find there to the office. What will doctors worry about when patients scan themselves, perform their own blood test and even genetic analysis at home? Will we able to persuade such patients to turn to doctors rather than trust algorithms? What if medical technology becomes so affordable and accurate that an algorithm with a simple home scan and blood test can reveal the health problems we face?

What if we started using augmented reality contact lenses that give us otherwise private information about the people we're looking at immediately? Kids born today represent the first generation for whom every life detail gets logged starting with a social security number assigned at birth. They generate sensitive information every second. Such big data sets can potentially improve healthcare, but how can we prevent companies and governments from using these against us, or to spy on us?

Services offering DNA sequencing directly to an individual raise serious questions. Do I own the data of my DNA, or does the company that makes it available to me? If I agree to let them use that information for research purposes, can I make sure that my DNA won't be revealed to my insurance company or employer? If I drink using a cup at a public place, and someone retrieves the cup with my DNA on it and uses that DNA for any purpose, can I do anything to prevent it?

In the wildest scenarios miniscule nanorobots coursing in our bloodstream could detect disease. These robots could send push notifications to our smartphones or digital contact lenses before the disease could develop. If microrobots in our body fluids become reality, how can we prevent terrorists from hacking them and controlling not only our health but our lives?

Terrorists in our time constantly attempt at stealing information and money. With disruptive innovations, health data and access to our body becomes another tempting target for them. We already have cases in which letters containing anthrax or other toxins have killed the recipient. With DIY biotechnology growing more popular, and molecular biology methods becoming cheaper, terrorists might just engineer their own agents in the same way that young geniuses engineer cells that brew beer in biotech competitions. The mundane can easily be made evil.

Without clear regulations and predetermined limits even small startups can pose a major threat. The biggest advantage of the current economy–the rise of startups– can lead to an enormous threat only because we don't know what they might create and how to keep it under control.

With the Internet of Things, where devices and our body are constantly connected, comes the Internet of Crime. Unless current security systems follow developments in software and hardware, we will either be in trouble or at least become suspicious of technological improvements, thinking perhaps that people could hack into our lives. Users of medical innovations who are unaware of the security gaps will make the job of terrorists easier. By sharing our precious health data over non–secure platforms, we invite them to use it against us.

According to a 2015 Forbes report, there were almost the same number of data breaches due to criminal attack than there were by lost or stolen computers and unintentional employee actions. When it comes to health technology, we pose the same risk to ourselves as criminals do.

There might even be new diseases in the future such as Nanotoxicological Shock or Cybernetic Septicemia. These would be characterized by the immunological reaction toward cybernetic body parts. If virtual reality becomes hardly distinguishable from reality, people might get addicted, leading to Dissociative Reality Disorder. When superintelligence arises, people could start boosting their cognitive abilities using genomics, smart drugs, and cybernetics. We might then end up with Superintelligence–induced Psychosis. If the rise of the robots yields unpleasant scenarios, Robophobia, the fear of robots, will spread.

At some point the data people generate and utilize will have to be tracked and analyzed in real time. We call this biosurveillance. The New York City Department of Health and Mental Hygiene developed a method after the 9/11 attacks to track the symptoms of those taken to emergency departments. The goal is to find patterns and detect bioterrorism attacks as soon as possible.

Our challenge is how much health information to reveal to the authorities that try to protect us. Even if authorities become able to protect us from data breaches, cyber attacks, and bioterrorism, we will need to remain cautious and conscious about what we do in the digital world. The preferred scenario is one in which I can protect myself by the methods I use on– and offline, and when my government assists me in doing that rather than taking decisions away from me.

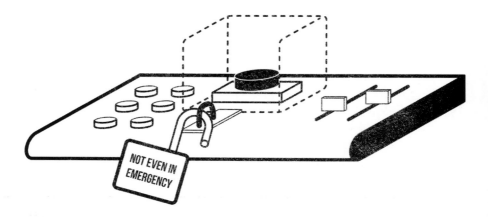

PART III. UPGRADING MY HEALTH

Witnessing the advances of technology through the eyes of a science fiction fan is amazing. But through conversations I have had with people from different backgrounds and countries, I have come to better understand why some are afraid of technological change. Their disquiet taught me to look at emerging healthcare from the perspective of a patient, policy maker, engineer, as well as a physician. Many times their perspectives challenged my own views. This forced me to convey my ideas more clearly.

What these discussions didn't take away was my fascination for innovative technology. When you see a paralyzed person walk again, a man who lost his arm grab a glass with a robotic prosthesis, the freedom wearable devices bestow, and witness how a supercomputer can organize hospital life in seconds then you see what technology is capable of. And we have seen nothing yet compared to what's to come.

From everyday health and sexuality to the future of humanity and the end of life, technology will change everything. Whether it happens for better or worse depends on us. We are the product of hundreds of millions of years of evolution, and we have just recently developed machines and algorithms to improve on that. Upgrading ourselves is inevitable.

By definition upgrading usually applies to technology, to material things. An upgrade is generally a replacement of hardware, software, or firmware with a newer or better version in order to bring the system up-to-date or improve its characteristics. No definition I am aware of mentions people even though we do have our own hardware we can upgrade by way of joint replacement and the like. The challenge we face is doing so in a way that we improve as humans instead of becoming technological extensions ourselves.

Upgrading health is not about fitness, six–packs, or running marathons. It is about living as healthily as possible in order to function as efficiently as possible. It includes physical, mental, and emotional health. All three elements are needed for a balanced life. We cannot wait for someone to change them. We need to do it ourselves.

No one should take the potential benefits of technology depicted in Part II for granted. Nothing will happen unless we as a society take charge. We are in a way building the largest pyramid ever built. One side of it is the need for better technology. Another side represents all the companies and developers creating these technologies. The third side is full of good regulations that foster this eco–system. The fourth side is our constant imagination for a better future without thinking of the limitations. One side can support the other one, and vice versa, as long as we have a high enough pyramid. At the apex sits human health, efficient medicine, and bright prospects. The blocks are available, but we haven't begun construction yet.

No system can be improved on without first understanding its elements and how they work together. The human body is the most complex system we know of. The central nervous system, hormone secretion, metabolic balance, digestion, and immunity are difficult to understand in detail, especially the molecular background behind them. What we can do, though, is to measure data points that have been proven useful in managing or predicting a given disease, and then adding additional data points with our new devices.

Doing so doesn't depend on money but on one's desire to improve health. What people get stuck on is the how. In the next sections, I will present the methods I have used for more than a decade.

WHICH DEVICE TO START WITH?

I get asked this a million times because people assume it is what they have to address first. But it isn't. Changing your life doesn't start with technology

First, answer the question, "Do you feel great?" Ask it every day and make sure the answer is yes. Read books with positive thoughts and repeat those thoughts daily. Find those time periods during which you are the most productive and defend them from any distraction. Make notes and plans every day, week, and month to make sure you are on track for the long term. This method will work for many, but not for all.

If you cannot identify problem areas with your lifestyle, then no device will help you. I knew I wanted to dedicate as much time as possible to those projects that made me happy, sleep better, and exercise daily. These were my starting points. You should get yours by asking the question above many times.

It is often said that 21 days are needed to form a new habit. This means if you do something every day for 21 days it will become a habit. People base this observation on a book called *Psycho–Cybernetics*. The author, Dr. Maxwell Maltz, who was a plastic surgeon in the 1950s, wrote that it takes about 21 days for his patients to adjust to a new nose or to the loss the phantom limb pain after an arm or leg was amputated. Today smartphone applications use a business model behind this 21 days rule. I have bad news. In the book, sold over 30 million copies, the author stated that "it requires a minimum of about 21 days for an old mental image to dissolve and a new one to jell". A minimum of 21 days. It means you still need to do the hard job yourself because doing the hard job can form a habit in your life.

When the new habit starts working, the goal is to withdraw the app and not to get dependent on it. Let's see what it looks like in practice.

When I started assigning scores between one and ten to my mental, physical, and emotional health I learned something about my lifestyle that I hadn't known before. I had a simple graph with numbers. Whatever issue you identify for yourself, I suggest you start with scoring. Say, for example, that your sleep is poor. For one week, assign a score from 1 to 10 to characterize how easily you woke up, and also log how many hours you slept. During the day give another score to how efficiently you function at work, and another rating for how tired you feel before turning in. You can tag days with noteworthy events, to help you remember what happened that day.

In one week you will have a cache of data. It takes 10 seconds every day to log these. There is no more efficient way. After looking through the data you can draw conclusions. You woke up really easily when you exercised the day before, or when you didn't have a heavy dinner. If you identify an issue that requires more detailed data that's the point at which technology can help.

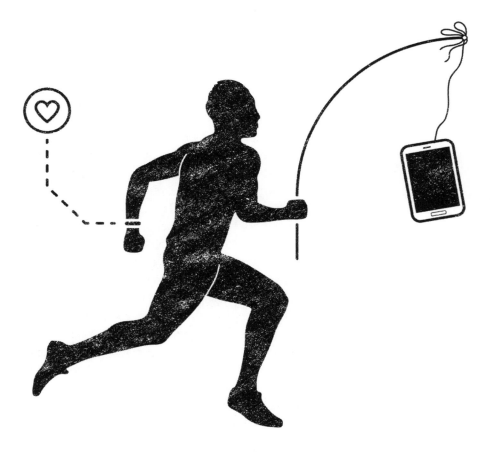

STEP BY STEP: SLEEP

We spend one third of our lives asleep. It affects how we feel, work, think, and socialize. Most people don't give any thought to the quality of their sleep. First, it never occurs to them, and secondly they don't know how. I discerned basic patterns about my sleep before I turned to technology. I knew I functioned best with 7 hours every day. Sleeping more than 8 hours and fewer than 6 both negatively affected my productivity. This is something you learn from simple observation. The reason I turned to a gadget to improve my sleep was another observation about seeing no particular reason how easily I can wake up. A lot of people suffer from the same.

I began using a Withings Pulse wristband during the night. It measured how much I moved around, how much time it took to fall asleep, and how long my deep sleep periods were. I used it nightly for two weeks while I kept a log of how easily I woke up and how energized I felt. Glancing at the graph I could tell what aspect of my sleep correlated with feeling energized. It wasn't total sleep time but rather having one long period of deep sleep. Let me repeat it: it didn't matter if I slept 6 or 8 hours when I had a single long deep–sleep period. It was quite a revealing piece of information.

Next was finding out what daily activities led to a lengthy deep sleep. Discovering this is trial and error. I began making notes about what I ate and drank before bedtime, whether it mattered when I exercised, used electronic devices, or read a book immediately before turning in. I discovered it was best to have dinner 3 hours before retiring if only to be properly hydrated. I saw that I didn't sleep well if I exercised in the evening, used electronic devices, and if wasn't equally tired mentally and physically. Every time I discovered a new correlation, I added it to my list, which became my personal guide to a good sleep.

Now I only measure sleep quality after a bad night's sleep, perhaps a few times a month to keep me on track. I solved my sleep problems, but I couldn't have done so without technology. One problem bothered me, though. I couldn't determine the best time to wake up every day because I couldn't monitor my sleep while I was asleep. But a smartwatch could.

I was an early adopter of the Pebble smartwatch, which awakens me with a gentle vibration. I know how much sleep I need and how to get that one long deep sleep. Now every night I need to make a decision about when to wake up. I cannot tell exactly when this is, but I allow some leeway to the free Morpheuz application on the smartwatch to decide. If I set my watch to wake me between 6:00 and 6:20 a.m., it will monitor my movements and try to find the best spot when it is easiest to awaken me. I'm not saying it finds it every single day, but most days I find it really easy to wake up at once when the smartwatch vibrates. So, two gadgets have changed the way I sleep and let me wake up ready to go.

I also tested the Fitbit to track sleep but it didn't provide enough details that I needed. The Checkme device measured blood oxygen levels during the night. It provided useful information, but was too big to wear comfortably. A smartphone app that many people use has you place it next to you on the pillow. It is supposed to monitor your sleep (it doesn't say how) and wake you up at the best time. For me, it was totally random, but everyone will have their own preference.

The reason I used devices that monitor health parameters under the mattress and wake me up with light and sound is that I don't want technology to control my sleep. I don't want to depend on a machine, but prefer my own decisions. I'm happy to fine tune my schedule if it leads to better sleep. But I want to do it myself.

STEP BY STEP: EXERCISE

When I fail to exercise, my mental performance decreases and my stress levels increase. This is another observation I have made over the years by looking at my scores. My need was simple: I wanted to find time and motivation to exercise every day. One was a bigger challenge than the other, but I found that gathering data can be a kind of motivation in itself. So I started measuring my daily activities.

I tried Striiv, which worked like Tamagotchi, the egg–shaped digital pet that millions used in the 1990s. I collected points by being physically active and built a world for my digital creature with them. It turned out to be too big and too uncomfortable. I then tried the Fitbit which gave me personal messages in addition to measuring the number of steps or floors I took, and calories burnt. I play football twice a week, otherwise run, and exercise at the gym or at home when I have no time for other activities.

I was curious about how active I was when I didn't do any of those. So I wore the FitBit when out of bed. I walked around while making phone calls to improve my step count. I took the stairs instead of escalators and elevators. After a few weeks I stopped using it but soon realized that I was still doing these beneficial things. The motivation had stuck. I still choose the stairs.

While running, I started wearing my smartphone in an armband. With the Runkeeper application I got useful data about my running sessions that included maps, pace, and elevation. By seeing when my friends went out for a run, I become motivated to do it even when I was having a hectic day.

As I pretty much hate running and find it incredibly boring, I tried another gadget, Wahoo Fitness. This in a chest strip measures my pulse while running. There are days when I need to run without becoming exhausted because I need to focus later in the day. Measuring my running pulse helps adjust to that. I can monitor it and slow down when needed. The report it provides after the session is amazingly detailed. I learned how much time I spent in power, anaerobic, aerobic, fat burn, and warm up modes. It feels like having a personal coach.

I also tried other applications that promise motivation. Zombies, Run, feeds me voice messages from virtual survivors around the world. I have to run away from zombies and find a hiding place. It sounds like a weird app, but you do run faster when you hear zombies chasing you. Imagine the same idea with augmented reality glasses.

Finding time to go out for a run can be a struggle. Sometimes my day is so full it becomes impossible. I still do pushups, and an app unsurprisingly called Push Ups helps me count how many I can do. It then designs a personal plan and tries to keep me practicing. With small tricks and a little time management, I exercise at least 25 days every month. Even when I have no opportunity to run, play football or go to the gym, I still can exercise at home or in a hotel room.

To save time I plan ahead for the next day. I never repeat the same exercise on two consecutive days in order to keep myself motivated. Instead of going for a long run, I sometimes take hundreds of stairs or do short sprints within the session. I make the whole process as exciting and diverse as possible. Nothing can stop me now.

STEP BY STEP: HEALTH CHECKUP

The Society of General Internal Medicine discourages physicians from performing "routine" tests in adults without any symptoms. One reason for this is cost–about $10 billion per year, which is more than the US spends on breast cancer.

We should not become addicted to logs and gadgets but enjoy a healthy life without constantly fiddling with them.

We shouldn't cut off those who like to monitor themselves from the healthcare system, but rather make doing so more efficient, cheaper, and more rational. If I want such a check up, I can send my ECG, pulse, blood pressure, oxygen saturation, and activity log to my doctor. If I need anything more thorough we can decide that without having to meet in person.

AliveCor tells me whether there are any abnormalities in my ECG. I can also ask remote specialists to check it. The Viatom Checkme device can do a daily checkup of ECG, pulse, and blood oxygen level, among other parameters. It interprets the results with a smiley which means I have nothing to do now. I'm hopeful that interpretation of the measured values will become much more sophisticated than that.

There is no reason to check my ECG every week, but being able to do so at home when I want is reassuring. I decided to measure only my blood pressure on a regular basis, twice a month. The relevant applications collect and visualize my data automatically.

Choosing the right device is a challenge. You might find the one device or online service that serves your need about a particular health issue, but there is always a better one. The best solution is not dealing with such measurements, but not all of us have that luxury. The job of making right choices among the myriad of opportunities is getting harder. The wearable marketplace on Amazon gets bigger every day. In an ideal world, patients who would like to take care of their health would not need to deal with it alone, but supported and advised by their physicians. This way, over–use and false positive misdiagnoses could be eliminated.

New applications and online services offer more and more. But which ones bring about a meaningful change in our lives? Check what stands behind the device. A CE or FDA approval helps one feel more favorable. Make sure the app is available for your device and whether its software is regularly updated. Comb through top reviews in the app store and ask the #wearables community on Twitter for what experience they have with it.

Choosing a health tracker should be an informed decision and you should find devices that best serve your needs. Some users buy tech for the sake of technology. Other trackers use them only when they need it. People who like competition want to beat their friends at every turn. Shy types need a tracker that motivates them to exercise. If you are a combination of these types, look for sophisticated devices.

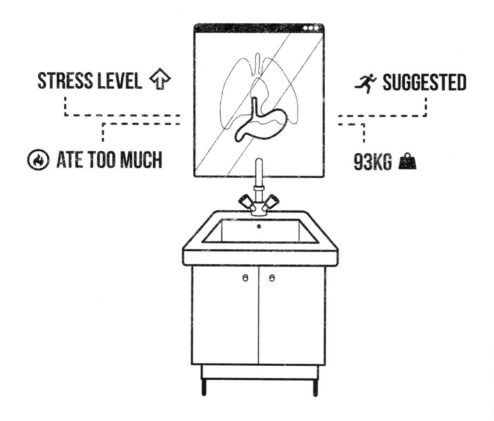

STRESS LEVEL ⬆

🏃 SUGGESTED

🔥 ATE TOO MUCH

93KG 🏋

STEP BY STEP: STRESS

The American Institute of Stress calls stress the number one health problem. A 2014 survey found that 77% of people have physical symptoms such as fatigue, headache, upset stomach, teeth grinding, and change in sex drive. While we have learned how to manage high blood pressure and diabetes, stress still eludes us.

Logging mental, physical, and emotional scores increased my awareness about the stress I felt daily. I discovered what habits made for a bad day, and I learned how to avoid them. I opened a Google document and assigned three scores to each date. This was the simplest digital solution, but now wearable devices make it easy to do it in a more sophisticated way.

Using the Tinké Zensorium device takes about 2 minutes. I put my thumb on its red lamp. It measures my pulse and oxygen saturation. Its algorithms calculate two scores between 1 and 99. One speaks to long-term cardiac fitness; the second to how stressed the user feels right now. It suggests how to change in order to get better scores. If the only reason I use it is to sit down for a few minutes and focus on breathing, then it is worth it.

The Pip device and its Loom application provide feedback about the user's stress level by measuring galvanic skin resistance. The app helps users calm down by having them make a cold and sad scene change into a warm and happy one. I see my stress level indicated by red, yellow or green buttons. I have learned ironically that if I focus on trying to reduce stress, I immediately make myself more stressed.

In addition to using external devices, consciously planning and monitoring my stress level is enormously useful. It helps, for example, if I work in advance. It means today I focus on projects which should be done by the same time next week. I still work many hours a day but my deadlines are never tonight. This mental flexibility removes most of the stress I would otherwise feel. It has worked for me, and I encourage you to find similar tricks that work for you.

STEP BY STEP: BRAIN

I wish I could have strengthened my cognitive skills when I was a medical student. Lumosity promises to do so with games backed by neuroscience. I must note that such claims are highly suspect, and so any "proof" claimed must be scrutinized with the utmost care. More than 50 games are claimed to improve mental flexibility, problem solving, focus, memory and speed in completing tasks. One game makes me drive more and more trains to their locations as fast as possible. Another one requires me to memorize patterns on a chess table. I have been playing these games since 2013, and I would not miss my daily dose. I haven't measured by scientific methods whether my cognitive skills have really changed, but when I need to completely focus on a project, I recall methods I learned while playing the games for better scores. Regular use seems to matter because self improvement is a marathon rather than a sprint.

When I want to relax I put on my Muse headband and open the related application on my smartphone. It guides me through the process of meditation. Then gives me feedback about how successful I was compared to myself before starting meditation. For example, I have to think of as many members of a category such as cars, books, or movies as I can in one minute. This is how it measures my active brain. Then I can set the length of the session and begin. The beach sound alone can make me relaxed, but I really start focusing on the reward, which is bird song. I couldn't do anything with an EEG graph therefore I need such a device to translate my EEG into digestible results. The app tells me when my brain was active or calm. This is the only distinction it can make. I've been meditating with it for over a year. And I can see how calm I mentally am while relaxing.

When I need to focus, I browse focusatwill.com and choose music types from lounge to up-tempo, which helps me focus for longer periods. Developers behind the freemium-based service checked the EEG signals of participants and filled the database only with the kind of music that supports focus. I switch to up-tempo when I need to work fast and to café creative when I need to come up with ideas.

To train myself how to reach a certain level of focus on purpose I use another headband, NeuroSky, and can see the results on my smartphone. I can fly a little Puzzlebox Orbit drone or a helicopter by tilting my phone after I have reached my desired level of focus. I thought the task would be easy, but controlling your focus deliberately is quite difficult. What helps me is counting backwards from 500 by 17 as quickly as I can. Imagine teaching future surgeons how to focus in long operating sessions with such a solution. A surgeon who practices focus is more likely and easily able to stay on task–the operation–than a surgeon who lives a life of relentless distraction.

THE DIGITAL JUNGLE

We cannot avoid the digital jungle when looking for advice about or devices to manage one's health. Social media, websites, and search engines connect us to each other and to good as well as faulty resources. If you need reliable advice, feeling comfortable in the digital world is crucial.

I use tricks called search operators on Google to save time and effort. When I need to find two words in the same query, I put AND between them. I use filetype:PDF to find only PDF documents. Instead of specifying PDF, I can use doc for Word documents, xls for spreadsheets, or any other file format. I do a search for "site:www.something.com treatment" when I only want to look for treatments on a specific website. Dozens of search operators can help me a lot to find what I need. If you don't find what you need on the first page of search results, you should probably try a new one instead of diving into the deep space of the Internet. If you want to get better at this, spend a few minutes on agoogleaday.com to learn by playing.

When the task is to find out more about the background of a particular health tracker, I do a search for its name: choose "Search tools" and click on past year in the "Any time" drop down menu. This way, I only get articles and news that mention the device during the past year, meaning that the information will be relatively current. I also do a search for the device on Twitter and Facebook to see what people are sharing about it, and to see what social media presence the company has. The more a company shares, the bigger the chance that it is not a scam.

When I need search results that will be identical for everyone globally, I use duckduckgo.com. This is a search engine that doesn't track its users' habits. When I have highly specific questions I go to wolframalpha.com. I do a search about what the weather was like on my birthday in the city where I was born, and it tells me. Or it can give me a plan about how much I have to exercise every week to lose weight.

I look for clues about quality on the company's website or social media channel by looking up author information, contact details, archives, privacy policy, disclaimer, and a clear description of what they do. I want to be sure that the company is real and that the information they provide is reliable. This helps me decide about their product.

It is also worth doing a quick search for either the device or the method it uses on Pubmed.com and scholar.google.com. These are databases of peer–reviewed biomedical papers, with Google Scholar being a bit better search engine. When a company claims that their method or product has been peer–reviewed, and that studies about its effectiveness are available, you can cross–check it in seconds on these two sites.

I have created automatic Google Alerts about those search queries I use regularly. Now whenever a new website, article, or announcement mentions my name, blog, or my favorite topics, I receive an e–mail notification. This is how I make sure that the Internet works for me rather than me having to go after new information.

I regularly follow about 500 medical websites, and don't have enough time to keep up with all of them. Instead I subscribe to their RSS feeds, meaning that new articles on that website are sent automatically to my RSS reader, Feedly.com. When I sit down to check my news, I decide which category to start with and which resource to check first. Every piece of information from my favorite websites comes to me. But I still receive hundreds of titles every day, and it's almost impossible to go through them all.

To prevent overload I fine tune my social media networks by deliberately selecting who I follow. When I check the top groups I follow on Tweetdeck.com and Facebook, I immediately see which articles will probably interest me that day. I use the groups on Linkedin, the hashtags on Twitter, and the communities on Google+ to address specific and relevant groups with my questions and ideas. Hundreds of thousands of assistants are working for me in the same way that I work for them.

Using search engines wisely, gathering information efficiently, and getting the most out of social media channels keeps me not only up–to–date but lets me enjoy the whole process. When it comes to the digital jungle we should feel at home just like Tarzan did.

WHAT ABOUT MEDICAL CONDITIONS?

I'm lucky not to have any major medical condition. At least, not yet. But an arsenal of medical devices is becoming available for a lot of ailments. Blood glucose trackers and related gadgets are available for diabetes. Devices can quantify the progress of asthma and the efficacy of treatment. A wearable smart bracelet, Empatica, can track epileptic seizures. Apps help kids comply with their therapy. The coming years will yield more devices for a range of medical conditions.

Choosing the right one can be a challenge. You should ask your doctor what they think about the device you are contemplating to help better manage your condition. If you are fortunate they will be up–to–date and have an opinion. If not, at least, you can explore this new direction together.

At some point everyone will face a major illness. The more we know about our health before it happens, the better we can manage it properly. If a physician discourages you for self–exploration, find another one. I had to find a GP and a health insurer who understand and value me being proactive.

Read blogs from respected authorities who deal with the health issue in question. Join online communities, and watch YouTube channels dedicated to them. Even in the case of rare diseases social media is full of relevant content. If for some surprising reason it is not, maybe it's time to support others by providing them with pieces of your own advice. Avoiding misleading and false information should be supported by medical professionals on this journey.

WHAT ARE THE NEXT UPGRADES?

By the time disruptive technologies become cheap and affordable everywhere, people will start embracing their benefits. This might mean that patients will measure any blood marker and vital sign at home, analyze their data through digital services, and use cognitive computers to help find the best diagnostic and therapeutic options. Does it sound like science fiction? Don't let our limited vision now lull us into underestimating our role in this. If patients can adjust to technological change and get the most out of it, medical professionals will do their best to maintain their current position in healthcare. They will have to improve constantly emphasizing the creativity of the human imagination and its power in making diagnoses and designing treatments by using algorithms utilizing big data as aids.

Investors might say that technology will replace most doctors eventually. I don't think this will happen. Even if technology were superior in diagnoses, most patients will still want human touch. If you could have an empathetic doctor or an algorithm that mimicked empathy, which would you choose?

Humans need interactions with other humans. In past centuries, doctors' work centered on dedication, commitment, and fulfillment. Today they face the unbidden reality of financial challenges, administrative headaches, and a huge amount of unshared responsibility. We made their job miserable. It's time to change that.

We could turn to social services to find motivations to live healthily, but frankly technology is simpler, more personalized, and affordable. As technology moves forward it is going to be even more so. You can pose your own questions about the future of medicine to communities on Twitter, Facebook, LinkedIn, and Google+. Many of us who are excited about the future are already there to help. Ask us, discuss, and debate.

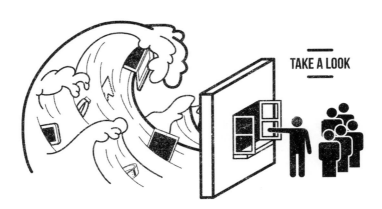

TAKE A LOOK

EXCITING WAVES ARE COMING

If we can build the pyramid I described before, the future is going to be really exciting. When things from robotic hands to novel cancer therapies become mainstream, more people will appreciate their potential to change lives. Economic demand for them will increase. We will have to work out ethical issues and regulations. I am optimistic because current trends all point into this direction.

Change in healthcare has been occurring for years. By around 2020 we will have access to devices that can measure anything. Wearables, inside-ables, and digestibles will appear with increasing frequency and people will become more accepting of them. The wearable revolution will have an effect on how we think and socialize.

The years 2015 to 2025 will see home testing become reality for simple blood analyses to complicated genome sequencing. A huge amount of data will appear, and we must rely on technology to make sense of it. Statisticians and biomedical engineers might rule during these years, when we will be able to customize treatment based on an individual's genomic background.

Between 2020 and 2030 robots and artificial intelligence will take center stage. These three eras will overlap in some aspects. The challenge will not be the pace of their development but our readiness to adopt them in practice. Hopefully, the principal overlap among these eras will be patient empowerment.

New technology often produces outcomes we can't prepare for. Industrialization prompted in labor unions and climate change. Software caused the need for firewalls and antivirus industries. The list could go on. Even the best technological evolution could lead to a world without privacy, freedom of choice, democracy, or even healthcare. It is not enough to improve technologies constantly; we have to adapt to whatever future we create.

Computers are amazing at completing specified tasks, and algorithms of artificial intelligence will make them able to respond to new situations and be creative. We cannot compete with computing power or their speed and scope. But if a robot or algorithm can take over your job, I believe it should do so. If your skills can be replaced with technology, you deserve it.

We need to find those skills such as creativity or problem solving we can maximally improve to the limits if there are any limits at all. Technology can actually help us in this, and there is no need to see ever–improving technology as a threat to society.

Only people with too much irrelevant information or with no information at all should be afraid. The era of the Internet has brought us information but hasn't taught us how to assimilate it and connect with knowledge. Acquire the skill of digital literacy and get ready for that. Don't expect technology to go away. It won't. Without technology there will be no healthcare at all. Without the Internet, billions of people are on their own regarding their health. Without telemedicine, distant villages will have no access to medical professionals. Without biotechnology, no new drug will come to market. More technology doesn't automatically lead to better care; we need get the most out of it, and we don't have this skill yet.

Computers make more efficient decisions if people are re–checking them. IBM's Watson doesn't make a decision by itself even though it checks more information in seconds than a doctor can in years. Surgical robots don't operate without human control in the way depicted in *Prometheus*. They augment what a surgeon can do. Wearable devices do not change our lifestyle, but give us the freedom to change it ourselves.

Disruptive technology coupled with the human brain is a winning combination. We should proudly stand atop our own inventions and observe, discover, and accomplish even more. By implementing new technology in our health and the practice of medicine, there will be no limits to what humanity can achieve.

ACKNOWLEDGEMENTS

This book would not exist without the constant support from my wife and my family. Running sessions, music from Focus@Will and some of the devices I use helped me find the best times to share my excitement in written form.

I'm grateful for those experts who were kind enough to dedicate time for answering my questions. Many thanks to Dr. Eric Topol, Chris Dancy, Dr. Danny Sands, Kerri Morrone Sparling, Jurriaan van Rijswijk, E-patient Dave deBronkart, Hugo Campos, Lucien Engelen, Dr. Jur Koksma, John Nosta, Professor Robert Langer, Professor Anthony Atala, Dr. Rafael Grossmann, John Sharp, Maria Konovalenko, Zoltan Istvan, Ian Pearson, Denise Silber and Dr. Larry Chu. Also I thank companies and organizations that shared their vision with me AliveCor, Withings, Tellspec, Scio, OpenBCI, Muse, Biobots, The Personalized Medicine Coalition, Intouch Health, MC10, Foodini, Organovo, and Ekso Bionics.

Without the questions audience members have asked me after my talks for over a decade, without their fascination or skepticism; there would only be empty pages.

REFERENCES

Part I. The Technological Revolution in Medicine
Losing faith in modern medicine
Journal of Patient Safety, A New, Evidence-based Estimate of Patient Harms Associated with Hospital Care http://journals.lww.com/journalpatientsafety/Fulltext/2013/09000/A_New,_Evidence_based_Estimate_of_Patient_Harms.2.aspx
National Center for Complementary and Integrative Health, What Complementary and Integrative Approaches Do Americans Use? https://nccih.nih.gov/research/statistics/NHIS/2012/key-findings
Can we see what is coming next?
Publicdomainreview.org, France in the year 2000 http://publicdomainreview.org/collections/france-in-the-year-2000-1899-1910/
Linear thinking http://dictionary.reference.com/browse/linear+thinking
The Best American Series: 20 Short Stories and Essays, Houghton Mifflin Harcourt (March 6, 2012)
It's time to upgrade our health
The Wall Street Journal, It Took the Telephone 75 Years To Do What Angry Birds Did in 35 Days. But What Does That Mean? http://blogs.wsj.com/economics/2015/03/13/it-took-the-telephone-75-years-to-do-what-angry-birds-did-in-35-days-but-what-does-that-mean/?mod=e2fb
Part II. The Most Exciting Questions About The Future Of Medicine
Chapter 1. Everyday Life
Why would you measure your ECG at home?
Forbes, 71% Of 16-To-24-Year-Olds Want 'Wearable Tech.' Why Don't I Even Want To Wear A Watch? http://www.forbes.com/sites/victorlipman/2014/09/22/71-of-16-24s-want-wearable-tech-why-dont-i-even-want-to-wear-a-watch/
Statista.com, Facts and statistics on Wearable Technology http://www.statista.com/topics/1556/wearable-technology/
Heart Rhythm, Using a novel wireless system for monitoring patients after the atrial fibrillation ablation procedure: the iTransmit study. http://www.ncbi.nlm.nih.gov/pubmed/25460854
Engadget, Can't decide on a wearable? Lumoid lets you try a box full of them http://www.engadget.com/2015/01/14/cant-decide-on-a-wearable-lumoid-lets-you-try-a-box-full-of-th

Bloomberg, Is Chris Dancy the Most Quantified Self in America? http://www.bloomberg.com/bw/articles/2014-06-05/is-chris-dancy-the-most-quantified-self-in-america

Vice.com, Forget the Apple Watch and Make Your Own Wearable Technology http://www.vice.com/read/forget-the-apple-watch-and-make-your-own-diy-wearable-technology-264

Will technology change the lives of people with diabetes?

Becoming Databetic, A Year in Diabetes Data http://databetic.com/?p=304

The University of Arizona, Smart Sox keep diabetics a step ahead of complications http://surgery.arizona.edu/in-the-news/smart-sox-keep-diabetics-step-ahead-complications-0

Will people measure vital signs at home?

Forbes, Obamacare Startup Oscar Health Hits A $1.5 Billion Valuation www.forbes.com/sites/stevenbertoni/2015/04/20/obamacare-startup-oscar-health-hits-a-1-5-billion-valuation/

Can technology really improve my sleep quality?

The American Sleep Association https://www.sleepassociation.org

Is it possible to scan food for ingredients?

WebMD, Allergies Health Center http://www.webmd.com/allergies/guide/food-allergy-intolerances

What would happen if patients led healthcare?

Acta Psychiatrica Scandinavica, Empowerment and satisfaction in a multinational study of routine clinical practice http://www.ncbi.nlm.nih.gov/pubmed/25471821

Health Informatics Journal, Empowering patients through social media: The benefits and challenges http://jhi.sagepub.com/content/20/1/50.short

Slate.com, The Heart of the Matter http://www.slate.com/articles/technology/future_tense/2015/03/patients_should_be_allowed_to_access_data_generated_by_implanted_devices.single.html

The BMJ, Lucien Engelen: Patients not included http://blogs.bmj.com/bmj/2013/08/16/lucien-engelen-patients-not-included/

Can I improve my brain?

Completed Research behind Lumosity www.lumosity.com/hcp/research/completed

Can social media help prevent and notify about epidemics?

BMJ Blog, Social media during epidemics: a poisoned chalice? http://blogs.bmj.com/bmj-journals-development-blog/2015/01/05/social-media-during-epidemics-a-poisoned-chalice/

Re/code, Seven Million People Used Facebook's Check-In Feature After Nepal Earthquake http://recode.net/2015/04/30/seven-million-people-used-facebooks-check-in-feature-after-nepal-earthquake/

Could we train doctors the way Duolingo teaches language?

Scandinavian Library Quarterly, Doctor's order: a tablet, digital course books and paperless curriculum http://slq.nu/?article=volume-47-no-2-2014-8#sthash.b95mtR58.dpuf

Will robots take over our jobs in healthcare?

IO9.com, Cool Experiment Puts Asimov's First Law Of Robotics To The Test io9.com/cool-experiment-puts-asimovs-first-law-of-robotics-to-t-1634921913

VentureBeat, Vinod Khosla says technology will replace 80 percent of doctors – sparks indignation http://venturebeat.com/2012/09/02/vinod-khosla-says-technology-will-replace-80-percent-of-doctors-sparks-indignation/

Business Insider, Experts predict robots will take over 30% of our jobs by 2025 – and white-collar jobs aren't immune http://www.businessinsider.com/experts-predict-that-one-third-of-jobs-will-be-replaced-by-robots-2015-5

The Atlantic, What Jobs Will the Robots Take? http://www.theatlantic.com/business/archive/2014/01/what-jobs-will-the-robots-take/283239/

When will we find the cure for cancer?

The National Cancer Institute www.cancer.gov

Will doctors always have to see patients in person?

The Wall Street Journal, A Fast Track to Treatment for Stroke Patients http://www.wsj.com/articles/a-fast-track-to-treatment-for-stroke-patients-1425338329

Philips.com, Philips tests innovative telehealth solution for pregnant women http://www.newscenter.philips.com/main/standard/news/press/2014/20140311-mobile-obstetrical-monitoring-project.wpd#.VaGAavlrjlV

MIT Technology Review, The Costly Paradox of Health-Care Technology http://www.technologyreview.com/news/518876/the-costly-paradox-of-health-care-technology/

Popularmechanics.com, 7 Medical Device Upgrades for Developing Countries http://www.popularmechanics.com/science/health/g456/7-medical-upgrades-for-developing-countries/?slide=1

Will innovative medical technology be accessible to the poor?

3dprintingindustry.com, e-NABLE & 3D Systems Push 3D Printed Prosthetics Even Further 3dprintingindustry.com/2015/06/11/e-nable-partners-with-3d-systems-to-push-3d-printed-prosthetics-even-further/

How will technology transform the future of sport?

Stanford Business, Five Trends Shaping the Future of Sports https://www.gsb.stanford.edu/insights/five-trends-shaping-future-sports

Chapter 2. Disruptive Trends
Can artificial food put an end to famine?

The World Food Programme, Hunger Statistics http://www.wfp.org/hunger/stats

Fortune, Here are some insane quotes about Elon Musk http://fortune.com/2015/05/11/elon-musk-book-ashlee-vance-quotes/

Singularity Hub, Robots Able to Pick Peppers, Test Soil, and Prune Plants Aim To Replace Farm Workers http://singularityhub.com/2014/07/14/pepper-picking-soil-testing-plant-pruning-robots-are-coming-to-farms/

Singularity Hub, Panel Tastes Lab-Grown Burger Made of Cultured Beef and Backed by Sergey Brin http://singularityhub.com/2013/08/05/panel-tastes-synthetic-lab-grown-burger-backed-by-sergey-brin/

Wired, Cow Milk Without the Cow Is Coming to Change Food Forever http://www.wired.com/2015/04/diy-biotech-vegan-cheese/

3dprintingindustry.com, 11 Food 3D Printers to Feed the Future 3dprintingindustry.com/2014/11/09/11-food-3d-printers/

National Geographic, Milk Grown in a Lab Is Humane and Sustainable. But Can It Catch On? http://news.nationalgeographic.com/news/2014/10/141022-lab-grown-milk-biotechnology-gmo-food-climate/

Wikipedia, Soylent https://en.wikipedia.org/wiki/Soylent_%28drink%29

NextBigFuture, Lab grown meat thirty thousand times cheaper than 18 months ago http://nextbigfuture.com/2015/05/lab-grown-meat-thirty-thousand-times.html

What comes after the wearable revolution?

Forbes, What Is The Future Of Fabric? These Smart Textiles Will Blow Your Mind http://www.forbes.com/sites/forbesstylefile/2014/05/07/what-is-the-future-of-fabric-these-smart-textiles-will-blow-your-mind/

The University of Tokyo, Fever alarm armband: A wearable, printable, temperature sensor : Professor Takao Someya, Department of Electrical Engineering and Information Systems http://www.t.u-tokyo.ac.jp/etpage/release/2015/150226_2.html

Given Imaging, PillCam http://www.givenimaging.com/en-int/innovative-solutions/capsule-endoscopy/pages/default.aspx

Proteus Health http://www.proteus.com/how-it-works/

Wikipedia, Radio-frequency identification https://en.wikipedia.org/wiki/Radio-frequency_identification#Hospitals_and_healthcare

Computer World, Office complex implants RFID chips in employees' hands http://www.computerworld.com/article/2881178/office-complex-implants-rfid-chips-in-employees-hands.html

IEEE, Know Your Wearables Slang spectrum.ieee.org/consumer-electronics/portable-devices/know-your-wearables-slang

Will we 3D print or grow organs?

The New Yorker, Print Thyself www.newyorker.com/magazine/2014/11/24/print-thyself

https://www.kidney.org/news/newsroom/factsheets/Organ-Donation-and-Transplantation-Stats

Gizmag, Organovo now selling tiny 3D-printed human livers http://www.gizmag.com/organovo-exvive3d-liver-models/34843/

Organovo.com, Organovo Describes First Fully Cellular 3D Bioprinted Kidney Tissue http://ir.organovo.com/news/press-releases/press-releases-details/2015/Organovo-Describes-First-Fully-Cellular-3D-Bioprinted-Kidney-Tissue/

Discover Magazine, Researchers' Quest for an Artificial Heart blogs.discovermagazine.com/crux/2015/06/02/artificial-heart/#.VaGli_IrjlX

BBC News, Whole organ 'grown' in world first http://www.bbc.com/news/health-28887087

Smithsonian Magazine, Soon, Your Doctor Could Print a Human Organ on Demand http://www.smithsonianmag.com/innovation/soon-doctor-print-human-organ-on-demand-180954951/#LWH2M3emrVP6MpGe.99

Vox Healthcare, An organ shortage is killing people. Are lab-grown organs the answer? http://www.vox.com/2014/11/20/7252365/lab-grown-organs

Can paralyzed people ever walk again?

Spinal Cord Injury (SCI) Facts and Figure https://www.nscisc.uab.edu/PublicDocuments/fact_figures_docs/Facts%202014.pdf

Science Magazine, Exoskeleton boot reduces cost of walking by 7% http://news.sciencemag.org/technology/2015/04/exoskeleton-boot-reduces-cost-walking-7

Fastcolabs.com, This Astonishing Robot-Inspired Prosthetic Promises Amputees An Easier Stride http://www.fastcolabs.com/3039714/this-astonishing-robot-inspired-prosthetic-promises-amputees-an-easier-stride

The New York Times, A new Approach For moving Robotic Arms With The

Brain http://www.nytimes.com/2015/05/26/science/a-new-approach-for-moving-robotic-arms-with-the-brain.html?_r=2

Should I get my genome sequenced?

Oxford Nanopore https://nanoporetech.com

Will the medical tricorder from Star Trek become real?

IEEE, The Race to Build a Real-Life Version of the "Star Trek" Tricorder spectrum.ieee.org/biomedical/diagnostics/the-race-to-build-a-reallife-version-of-the-star-trek-tricorder

Wikipedia, Medical Tricorder https://en.wikipedia.org/wiki/Medical_tricorder

Why are supercomputers still not used in healthcare?

Singularity Hub, Infographic: Trillion-Fold Rise in Computing Puts a 1985 Supercomputer on Our Wrists singularityhub.com/2015/05/25/infographic-trillion-fold-rise-in-computing-puts-a-1985-supercomputer-on-our-wrists/

Popular Science, How Supercomputing Is Cracking The Mysteries Of Human Origins http://www.popsci.com/how-supercomputing-cracking-mysteries-humankinds-origins

Ars Technica, University builds cheap supercomputer with Raspberry Pi and Legos http://arstechnica.com/information-technology/2012/09/university-builds-cheap-supercomputer-with-raspberry-pi-and-legos/

Could doctors literally look through patients?

Medgadget, EyeSeeMed Lets Surgeons Browse Patient Data With Their Eyes (VIDEO) www.medgadget.com/2014/11/eyeseemed-lets-surgeons-browse-patient-data-with-their-eyes-video.html

Philips.com, Experience the future of wearable technology http://www.healthcare.philips.com/main/about/future-of-healthcare/

Bionicly, 8 Ways Google Glass is Disrupting Health bionicly.com/8-ways-google-glass-is-disrupting-health/

Science Alert, New bionic contact lenses could make glasses obsolete http://www.sciencealert.com/new-bionic-contact-lenses-could-make-glasses-obsolete

Is printing out medical equipment cheaper than manufacturing?

http://www.mddionline.com/article/fdas-view-3-d-printing-medical-devices

Fierce Medical Devices, Stratasys, Worrell partner for faster, cheaper 3-D printed medical devices http://www.fiercemedicaldevices.com/story/stratasys-worrell-partner-faster-cheaper-3-d-printed-medical-devices/2014-10-31

Medicalplasticsnews.com, Silicone breast prostheses 50% cheaper to make with 3D printing http://www.medicalplasticsnews.com/technology/silicone-breast-prostheses-50-cheaper-to-make-with-3d-printing/

inside3dp.com, The medical world could become much cheaper thanks to 3D printing http://www.inside3dp.com/medical-world-become-much-cheaper-thanks-3d-printing/

Will we ever treat individuals based on their own DNA?

MIT Technology Review, Internet of DNA www.technologyreview.com/featuredstory/535016/internet-of-dna

MIT Technology Review, Google Wants to Store Your Genome www.technologyreview.com/news/532266/google-wants-to-store-your-genome/

MIT Technology Review, Genome Study Predicts DNA of the Whole of Iceland www.technologyreview.com/news/536096/genome-study-predicts-dna-of-the-whole-of-iceland/

For how long will we test drugs on actual people?

The Economist, Towards a body-on-a-chip www.economist.com/news/science-and-technology/21654013-first-organ-chips-are-coming-market-and-regulators-permitting-will-speed

Wyss Institute, Organs-on-Chips wyss.harvard.edu/viewpage/461/

What will hospital of the future look like?

Ochsner news, Ochsner's O Bar Uses Interactive Health Technology to Enhance Patient Engagement news.ochsner.org/news-releases/ochsners-o-bar-uses-interactive-health-technology-to-enhance-patient-engage/

Will virtual reality take over our lives?

Medhacker, Interventional Cardiologist Explores Virtual Reality in Medical Procedures with Jaunt VR http://medhacker.com/2015/05/02/interventional-cardiologist-explores-virtual-reality-in-medical-procedures-with-jaunt-vr/

Forbes, How Virtual Reality May Change Medical Education And Save Lives www.forbes.com/sites/robertglatter/2015/05/22/how-virtual-reality-may-change-medical-education-and-save-lives/

GestureTek, Gesture-Based Virtual Reality Systems for Improved Results in Rehabilitation and Therapy www.gesturetekhealth.com/products-rehab.php

Wikipedia, Video Game Addiction https://en.wikipedia.org/wiki/Video_game_addiction

Will there be operating rooms manned only with robots?

Robot Draws Blood https://www.youtube.com/watch?v=s30FPobi9iA

Brown University, History Of Robotic Surgery biomed.brown.edu/Courses/BI108/BI108_2004_Groups/Group02/Group%2002%20Website/history_robotic.htm

The Wall Street Journal, The Pros and Cons of Robotic Surgery www.wsj.

com/articles/SB10001424052702304655104579163430371597334

MIT Technology Review, Security Experts Hack Teleoperated Surgical Robot www.technologyreview.com/view/537001/security-experts-hack-teleoperated-surgical-robot/

The Wall Street Journal, Google Moves to the Operating Room in Robotics Deal With J&J blogs.wsj.com/digits/2015/03/27/google-moves-to-the-operating-room-in-robotics-deal-with-jj/

Can an algorithm diagnose better than a doctor?

Wikipedia, Advanced Chess https://en.wikipedia.org/wiki/Advanced_Chess

IBM.com, IBM Watson Health, Epic and Mayo Clinic to Unlock New Insights from Electronic Health Records https://www-03.ibm.com/press/us/en/press-release/46768.wss

Chapter 3. And Beyond
Will we be able to transmit or read thoughts?

Listverse, 10 Astounding Medical Achievements http://listverse.com/2013/04/22/10-astounding-medical-achievements/

Wikipedia, Kevin Warwick https://en.wikipedia.org/wiki/Kevin_Warwick#Deep_brain_stimulation

Scientific American, 100 Trillion Connections: New Efforts Probe and Map the Brain's Detailed Architecture www.scientificamerican.com/article/100-trillion-connections/

Aeon.co, Do we really want to fuse our brains together? aeon.co/magazine/psychology/do-we-really-want-to-fuse-our-minds-together/

Top500.org, The Race to Build the World's Greatest Supercomputer www.top500.org/blog/the-race-to-build-the-worlds-greatest-supercomputer/

Deepstuff.org, The Coming Merge of Human and Machine Intelligence Read more at http://www.deepstuff.org/the-coming-merge-of-human-and-machine-intelligence/#IK6ze2Ljm9lrGPBI.99 www.deepstuff.org/the-coming-merge-of-human-and-machine-intelligence/

IEEE, Organic Electrochemical Transistors for Reading Brain Waves spectrum.ieee.org/tech-talk/biomedical/devices/organic-electrodes-read-brainwaves-

What makes someone a cyborg?

Telegraph, The Real Cyborgs s.telegraph.co.uk/graphics/projects/the-future-is-android/index.html

What is a Cyborg? https://ethics.csc.ncsu.edu/risks/ai/cyborgs/study.php

Nick Bostrom, Ethical Issues in Human Enhancement www.nickbostrom.com/

ethics/human-enhancement.html

Wikipedia, Texting while driving https://en.wikipedia.org/wiki/Texting_while_driving

What is the secret to a long life?

Wikipedia, Alameda County Study https://en.wikipedia.org/wiki/Alameda_County_Study

The Okinawa Study www.okicent.org/cent.html

The Huffington Post, Outpaced by Innovation: Canceling an XPRIZE www.huffingtonpost.com/peter-diamandis/outpaced-by-innovation-ca_b_3795710.html

What would happen to society if we all lived beyond 130?

European Stakeholder involvement in Ageing society www.pacitaproject.eu/ageing-society/

Pew Research Center, Living to 120 and Beyond: Americans' Views on Aging, Medical Advances and Radical Life Extension www.pewforum.org/2013/08/06/living-to-120-and-beyond-americans-views-on-aging-medical-advances-and-radical-life-extension/

Wikipedia, Aging of Japan https://en.wikipedia.org/wiki/Aging_of_Japan

Scienceroll, 9 Ways Technology Helps Manage Alzheimer's and Parkinson's Disease scienceroll.com/2015/03/18/9-ways-technology-helps-manage-alzheimers-and-parkinsons-disease/

Wikipedia, Life Expectancy https://en.wikipedia.org/wiki/Life_expectancy#mediaviewer/File:Life_Expectancy_at_Birth_by_Region_1950-2050.png

The Atlantic, What Happens When We All Live to 100? www.theatlantic.com/features/archive/2014/09/what-happens-when-we-all-live-to-100/379338/

Should I get cryopreserved when I die?

BBC, Episode 3: Extending Lives www.bbc.com/specialfeatures/horizons-business/seriesfive/episode-3-extending-lives/?vid=p02rwp1y

BBC, Human hibernation: Secrets behind the big sleep http://www.bbc.com/future/story/20140505-secrets-behind-the-big-sleep

Wikipedia, Anna Bågenholm https://en.wikipedia.org/wiki/Anna_Bågenholm

Wikipedia, Cryonics https://en.wikipedia.org/wiki/Cryonics#Legal_issues

Will nanorobots swim in our bloodstream?

IEEE, Medical Microbots Take a Fantastic Voyage Into Reality spectrum.ieee.org/robotics/medical-robots/medical-microbots-take-a-fantastic-voyage-into-reality

Scientific American, Nanobots Start to Move www.scientificamerican.com/

article/nanobots-start-to-move/

Gizmag, Scallop microbots designed to swim through your bodily fluids www.gizmag.com/scallop-microbots-swim-body-max-planck/34589/

Wikipedia, Nanobiotechnology https://en.wikipedia.org/wiki/Nanobiotechnology

NextBigFuture, Pfizer partnering with Ido Bachelet on DNA nanorobots nextbigfuture.com/2015/05/pfizer-partnering-with-ido-bachelet-on.html

Foresight Institute, A Practical NanoRobot for Treatment of Various Medical Problems www.foresight.org/Conference/MNT8/Papers/Rubinstein/index.html

Why are futurists usually wrong about healthcare?

Wikipedia, Predictions made by Ray Kurzweil https://en.wikipedia.org/wiki/Predictions_made_by_Ray_Kurzweil#2019

Should we be afraid of artificial intelligence in medicine?

Gizmodo, The AI Revolution: How Far Away Are Our Robot Overlords? gizmodo.com/the-ai-revolution-how-far-away-are-our-robot-overlords-1684199433

How does technology change sexuality?

The Daily Dot, The future of virtual sex is like nothing you've ever felt before www.dailydot.com/technology/future-of-virtual-sex-kiiroo-fleshlight-oculus-porn/

The Hug Shirt http://cutecircuit.com/the-hug-shirt/#after_full_slider_1

The Independent, iOS 9: iPhone will now track sexual activity www.independent.co.uk/life-style/gadgets-and-tech/news/ios-9-iphone-will-now-track-sexual-activity-10307408.html

Send A Kiss Over The Internet With The Kiss Transmission Device https://youtu.be/PspagsTFvIg

The Huffington post, Soon, Your Sex Doll Will Have An Intelligent Conversation With You www.huffingtonpost.com/2015/06/11/sex-doll-talks-back-real-doll_n_7563764.html?ir=Technology&ncid=fcbklnkushpmg00000063

Davecat futuristmm.com/futurist-spotlight/davecat/

The Wall Street Journal, The Future of Virtual Sex www.wsj.com/articles/the-future-of-virtual-sex-1423845474

What if people want to replace healthy body parts for prosthetics?

The Alternative Limbs Project http://www.thealternativelimbproject.com/types/alternative-limbs/

How can we prevent bioterrorism from hijacking innovations?

Forbes, Why Medical Identity Theft Is Rising And How To Protect Yourself www.forbes.com/sites/laurashin/2015/05/29/why-medical-identity-theft-is-rising-and-how-to-protect-yourself/

IEEE, Hackers Invade Hospital Networks Through Insecure Medical Equipment spectrum.ieee.org/view-from-the-valley/biomedical/devices/hackers-invade-hospital-networks-through-insecure-medical-equipment

Wikipedia, Bioterrorism, https://en.wikipedia.org/wiki/Bioterrorism

IO9.com, 10 Diseases That Might Afflict Us In The Future io9.com/10-diseases-that-might-afflict-us-in-the-future-1666688319

Part III. Upgrading My Health

The Huffington Post, How Long Does It Actually Take to Form a New Habit? (Backed by Science) http://www.huffingtonpost.com/james-clear/forming-new-habits_b_5104807.html

Choosing Wisely, Society of General Internal Medicine http://www.choosing-wisely.org/societies/society-of-general-internal-medicine/

NPR.org, Maybe You Should Skip That Annual Physical http://www.npr.org/sections/health-shots/2015/04/06/397100748/maybe-you-should-skip-that-annual-physical

The American Institute of Stress, "People are disturbed not by a thing, but by their perception of a thing." http://www.stress.org/daily-life/

Wikipedia, Upgrade https://en.wikipedia.org/wiki/Upgrade

Focus@Will music effects on brain electrical activity and brain function https://www.focusatwill.com/wp/wp-content/uploads/2013/04/White-Paper-on-Focus@Will-Reading-Research.pdf

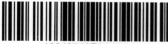

16640740R00120

Printed in Great Britain
by Amazon